The Humor Revolution

Dr. Alice Presents

The Humor Revolution

Laugh More. Stress Less.

Alice Glasser, MD, MPH

iUniverse, Inc.
New York Bloomington Shanghai

The Humor Revolution
Laugh More. Stress Less.

iUniverse books may be ordered through booksellers or by contacting:

iUniverse
1663 Liberty Drive
Bloomington, IN 47403
www.iuniverse.com
1-800-Authors (1-800-288-4677)

Because of the dynamic nature of the Internet, any Web addresses or links contained in this book may have changed since publication and may no longer be valid.

The views expressed in this work are solely those of the author and do not necessarily reflect the views of the publisher, and the publisher hereby disclaims any responsibility for them.

ISBN: 978-0-595-49536-8 (pbk)
ISBN: 978-0-595-61141-6 (ebk)

Printed in the United States of America

To Frio

My Loving Laugh Partner

Contents

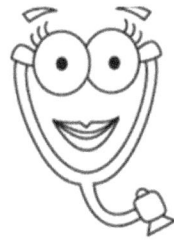

Laughing with Dr. Alice
Experience the Power of Joy

1. The Feel Good Lifestyle

She was still in a deep sleep when the radio erupted with the oldies tune *I think I'm going out of my head.* "Now there's a song that's still not dated," she thought as she sat up and slid her feet into her new slippers made of sustainable sheepskin and recycled pizza boxes. She then pitter pattered into the kitchen. It was time for her usual morning bowl of *Fiberlicious.*

It was, of course, a whole grain cereal made of flaxseed, organic oat bran and macrobiotic wheat germ that she mixed with fat-free, calcium enriched soymilk. The key to eating this fiber feast was simple: ingest it quickly or else the spoon gets stuck in the glue-like mass. This was not, perhaps, the most appetizing of breakfasts, which is why she deserved a mouth-watering reward after eating it. So every week she went to a fabulous French bakery and bought a few chocolate croissants. Okay, so maybe she bought more like a dozen. They do freeze well, right? And she did need that one small taste of buttery chocolate heaven after finishing her cereal, didn't she? Of course, there were a few mornings when she took that tiny bite of heaven first and then ended up eating the whole croissant ... and then another. Well, to be honest, she couldn't even remember the last time she actually ingested any *Fiberlicious.* But that wasn't a problem. Think of all those calories she avoided everyday. What a great way to watch one's weight.

Breakfast was not the only item she needed to ingest. Her doctor had given her a prescription to lower her borderline cholesterol since she was supposed to try to achieve one of society's latest goals: Immortality. Everyone knows that *Ninety is the New Twenty*, right?

However, she was having a bit of a problem with her prescribed immortality drug. It made her muscles ache to the point that her doctor added a non-steroidal pain killer. Unfortunately, this pill really upset her stomach. Between pain and nausea, being twenty again quickly lost its appeal, so her doctor suggested that she stop both meds for a while and proposed a more natural route for her longevity. "Just watch your fats," he said, "and consider taking some omega-threes. You can find them at pharmacies or health food stores."

Watch her fats? Her doctor made it sound like all she had to do was place her olive oil, peanut oil, and canola oil on the counter top so she could 'watch' them every time she came into the kitchen. And that wasn't all. She could also open the fridge anytime she wanted to 'watch' the butter lazily lounging on its dish. But that wasn't what the doctor meant, was it? No, she was supposed to start putting limits on how much and what kind of fat she ingested.

She wasn't too happy about limiting her croissant intake, so she decided to go see the Wellness Consultant at her local health food store and ask about omega threes.

"Omega threes are good fats," said the consultant.

"Good fats?" she asked puzzled. "As opposed to bad fats?"

"Exactly," said the consultant.

"Who gets to decide this?" she asked. "Is there a fat czar?"

"No, but scientific studies have suggested that some fats are bad for your heart, while others actually protect it, like the omega threes."

"Is this a widely accepted belief?" she asked.

"We think so," said the consultant.

"You only think so? Does that mean that omegas are one of those red or blue issues?"

"Red or blue?"

"Exactly," she said. "Which party endorses them?"

"Ma'am? I don't understand you."

"I am simply asking if either major political party endorses them. Is there a pro or con omega faction?"

"Ma'am, they are just fats, not a hot political issue."

"Okay, then why don't you just tell me how I take them," she said.

"They come in fish oil pills."

"Fish oil pills? How ... unappealing," she said while thinking the word unappealing doesn't even begin to describe a fish oil pill. At least she had finally discovered an "edible something" that made *Fiberlicious*, even with a spoon stuck in it, look like it belonged on the cover of Martha Stewart's next book. She sighed big time. Why couldn't omega threes come in chocolates or caramels or better yet deep-fried? Why did anything that was "good for you" have to be unpleasant or down-right icky? Had both houses of Congress, unbeknownst to her, added that resolution as the Twenty-Third Amendment to the U.S. Constitution?

The consultant tried to reassure her. "You don't taste or smell the fish. You just swallow the pills."

Just swallow the pills? Obviously the consultant had never tried to take fish oils. The pungent aroma of fishy fumes almost knocked her out when she opened the bottle for the first time. Fortunately, there was an easy solution to the problem. She simply never opened the bottle again.

After breakfast, she made her way into the bathroom where she momentarily froze. Wait. There was no need to panic. Her scale was broken. Of course, it was a bit annoying that her high tech *Talking Scale* had ceased to function after only one month. And she really didn't think that it had anything to do with that morning when she got a bit frustrated with the deep, male computer voice saying: *You weigh such and such pounds today. You should only weigh such and such.* She hadn't whacked it that many times with the large, hard toilet bowl plunger, had she?

And she was definitely going to buy another scale soon, because watching your weight is so important, right? In fact, she had already tried to purchase another one, but she just couldn't find what she wanted, even after asking for help.

"I'm looking for a scale," she had inquired.

"Any particular kind?" asked the salesperson.

"The kind that measures in ounces."

"You're in luck!" he said. "We do carry a scale that measures ounces as well as pounds! They are …"

"No, no. I want one that only measures ounces. I want to be able to tell my friends that I lost 50 big ones in just a month," she said.

"Ma'am, they don't make that type of scale."

"Why not?"

"I don't know."

"Well, they should," she said. "Here's my card. When you start selling that kind, call me, okay?"

Well, she was still waiting to hear, but meanwhile, she did step on that broken scale every day and tried to sense her weight. And guess what? This method seemed to be working because she felt thinner and that's what really matters, isn't it? And it's not like she wasn't exercising to try to keep her weight down. She had bought quite an expensive pair of athletic shoes that frankly, after reading all the claims about them, might just be the answer to world peace. Hadn't the manufacturers promised that these shoes would bring a peace and comfort to her body that she had never known? And they did feel great, but she also knew that the more she wore them, the sooner they would wear out. She couldn't afford another pair for a very long time. So she just kept them in her closet in the shoebox. She was pleased to note that after months of ownership, the shoes still looked new. Besides, who wants to go out jogging in the midst of a Buffalo winter and face the bitter cold, the ice, or the snowdrifts? Not her. Of course she lived in Los Angeles, but that's almost the same thing, isn't it?

Fortunately, there was an indoor alternative. She could work out on the exercise machine currently residing in her bedroom. Aerobic exercise was only part of the picture, right? She also understood the importance of weight bearing exercises since every middle-aged woman needed to strengthen her muscles and, more importantly, her bones. Why? Well, we now know that 100 years ago every woman over the age of 50 apparently died of a broken hip. What makes this particularly interesting is that no one noticed all these women falling and dying at the time, but that doesn't seem to matter. What matters is building up one's bones so she decided to do a full work out tomorrow. And if not then, definitely the next day. For sure by next year. Maybe by then she would've adjusted to her work out machine that was apparently designed by someone with a PhD in the torture methods of the Spanish Inquisition. Of course she should have figured this out sooner. After all, her apparatus is called *The Rack*. And besides, she was not too enthused about changing into her new hand woven organic cotton work out clothes because they were just the tiniest bit itchy. Actually, they were more than a bit itchy. Had they had been designed by someone who loves to burrow in a red anthill with a porcupine? She didn't want to irritate her sensitive, aging skin, did she?

At least there was one thing she didn't have to worry about: smoking. She had never smoked and never planned to. That could be the ace in her pocket when she saw her new doctor today. She'll just make sure the conversation goes like this:

Dr: Are you taking the medication prescribed?

Her: No, I'm taking a small vacation from it, but I don't smoke.

Dr.: Have you thought about losing some weight?

Her: I think about it every day when I step on my broken scale, but I don't smoke. I never have.

Dr.: Are you exercising regularly?

Her: I have a whole exercise program worked out that I do plan to try by next year, but I never light up. In fact, I have never even inhaled second hand smoke.

And if that plan of distraction didn't work, her new HMO's delivery approach might just save her. She had found out that every doctor in her new plan had to see 100 patients a day. Four minutes a pop doesn't exactly give anyone much time for berating. Wait. I meant counseling, of course.

So you can imagine her surprise when a very relaxed, middle-aged woman appeared who, after introducing herself as Dr. Alice, began to chit and chat and smile and laugh.

Her patient finally had to ask: "Don't you have a lot of people to see today?"

"Not at all," she said. "The rest of my patients cancelled, all 99 of them. I can spend all day with you. So, what's on your mind?"

It all came pouring out: glue for breakfast, fish oil pills that obliterate olfactory nerves, frostbite from jogging in the bitter cold of Los Angeles, and let's not forget, working out to one's own screams of pain. Wasn't there something she could do for her body that didn't make her feel like she was being sacrificed on the altar of health?

"Actually, there is," said Dr. Alice. "You can smile and laugh more."

"I can smile and laugh more?"

"Or giggle and guffaw. It's your choice."

"Excuse me," she said, feeling somewhat offended, "I am not joking about this."

"Neither am I," said Dr. Alice. "Humor is not a laughing matter. It can make such a significant contribution to your mental and physical health that I believe the lack of humor in peoples' lives to be a public health problem. And I am not alone in making this observation. There's a whole movement backed by scientific data to support this viewpoint."

"Are you telling me in all seriousness that there are scientists studying humor?" she asked.

"Yes! It's estimated that right now, as we speak, more than 200 researchers worldwide are looking into humor and how it affects our health."

"I had no idea," she said.

"And that's why I want to tell you about it. Even a simple laugh can cause such an amazing cascade of physical and mental health effects that I believe the moment is ripe for a Humor Revolution!"

"A Humor Revolution?"

"A Humor Revolution is about laughing more and stressing less. It's time for people to actively seek out humor and laughter for the benefit of their minds, bodies and pure enjoyment. And, just as importantly, they also need to realize that they don't have to spend so much time running around stressed out as if they are over caffeinated and in need of a teddy bear to hug."

"That's a funny image," she said.

"But it's true, isn't it?"

"I'm afraid so."

"And we don't need to live our lives like this. We can choose to smile and laugh more."

"But can a Humor Revolution happen?" she asked.

"Why not? Just arm the masses with Weapons of Laugh Instruction while health care workers unite, stand up and shout: Giggle or Die!"

That comment almost caused her to stand up as she asked: "Are you sure that's what you want to shout?"

"Well, maybe I need to shout this instead: It's time for humor to be taken as seriously as diet, exercise or any other Lifestyle Choices that make important contributions to our health. There are many scientific studies to support this claim including an especially telling one conducted by Dr. George Valliant, a Professor of Psychiatry at Harvard. He has followed a group of people for more than 60 years and has found that seven Lifestyle Choices lead to emotional and physical health if practiced before the age of 50.[1] Would you like to try to guess them?"

"Sure," she said. "I think I'll start with diet."

"No."

"Not diet?" she asked totally amazed.

"No."

"You're kidding?"

"No, I am not!"

A wave of pure joy passed over her as she imagined pouring that box of Fiberlicious down the sink. Wait. Not the sink. That might permanently clog her pipes. Maybe she could use it for kitty litter? She was still congratulating herself on a great recycling idea when she heard Dr. Alice say: "But one of the Lifestyle Choices is related to diet."

"Weight?"

"Yes, any other guesses?"

"How about exercise and not being a smoker?"

"You got three," said Dr. Alice.

"Alcohol?"

"Yes, however you don't need to think prohibition, just minimal intake. That's four."

"It's getting harder," she said. "Maybe you should give me hint."

"Okay, what if I say for better or for worse?"

"Marriage?"

"It seems to keep people healthier and so does my BS," said Dr. Alice.

"Your own BS helps keep you healthy?" she asked.

"I was referring to my Bachelor of Science degree."

"So a higher education level makes a difference?"

"It does and finally, there is one last Lifestyle Choice that should be obvious since it's what started this whole conversation."

"Humor?"

"Yes, using humor to cope with life," said Dr. Alice. "And that's not BS because Lifestyle Choices have a tremendous impact on our health and on our longevity. Studies have suggested that genes alone determine less than 3% of anyone's life span.[2] How you choose to live your life is probably the most important factor in determining how long you live."

"That's fascinating and yet, it's rather intimidating to think that I have so much power over my own life."

"That's one way to look at it, but isn't it also exciting to think that by simply smiling and laughing more, you may live longer? Isn't that empowering and appealing?"

"That does sound appealing," she said.

"Of course it's appealing which is why I call humor The Feel Good Lifestyle. It differs from the other Lifestyle Choices because humor comes with usual physical benefits plus an unusual mental one: a jolt of joy that immediately enhances the quality of your life. And don't ever undervalue the importance of enjoying life."

"I agree that life is best enjoyed, yet I'm still wondering, why I have never heard of humor referred to as a Lifestyle Choice before?"

"That's a good question," said Dr. Alice.

"When people say that," she said, "it usually means there is no answer."

"Let's just say there aren't any widely accepted answers, but I have several ideas if you want to hear them."

"I am curious."

"I'm afraid that I have to start with a somewhat cynical take, even though I don't consider myself a pessimist. However, from the perspective of a drug company or any other health vendor, there is just no money to be made from humor. There is no pill that can be advertised on your television screen every fifteen minutes. There isn't even a food to push or any equipment to market."

"That's too bad," she said. "I would much rather have to watch an ad extolling a humor pill than what we currently have to watch: constant plugs for either restless leg or irritable bowel syndrome."

"And the food situation is not much better," said Dr. Alice. "One article comes out extolling cinnamon as a way to lower cholesterol and the next thing I see are supermarket shelves lined with everything from cinnamon cereal to cinnamon cheese. However, not being able to market humor is not the only reason why so few people know about its benefits. I also believe we're just not used to taking humor seriously and we're especially not used to thinking of humor as a serious health problem."

"That's true."

"And what makes this even trickier is that we usually equate Lifestyle Choices with some kind of suffering or sacrifice. Telling people to start chuckling more doesn't fit in with these expectations, does it?"

"No it doesn't," she said.

"Fortunately, there is now a movement fostered by caring professionals to spread the word about humor and health. To help people take this message more seriously they have coined the term Therapeutic Humor. If you think about it, no other Lifestyle Choice uses any qualifying word. Have you ever heard anyone mention Therapeutic Exercise or Therapeutic Marriage?"

"No, but it might be a good idea," she said. "People might put more thought into tying the knot if we called it Therapeutic Marriage."

"Feel free to start using it," said Dr. Alice. "Who knows? Maybe we'll soon start receiving wedding invitations that read: *Joe & Jane Giggle invite you to attend the Therapeutic Marriage of ...*"

"Or how about: *Come join us in sun-drenched Jamaica as we celebrate the Therapeutic Marriage of ...*"

"Send me the invite to that one," said Dr. Alice. "However, I do want to make one thing clear: Therapeutic Humor has nothing to do with reclining in some shrink's office spending hours and hours analyzing bad knock, knock jokes from childhood. It's not a formal type of therapy used by psychologists to help people with depression or other mental issues. It may not even be appropriate under those circumstances. Therapeutic Humor is about using humor and laughter to promote health, wellness and the enjoyment of life through a better appreciation of the absurdities that flourish everywhere."

"So Therapeutic Humor can be many things?" she asked.

"It can be anything that makes you smile because it's an entire spectrum of laughs. You can experience it alone, like taking the time to watch your favorite funny DVD or with others as in playing a fun game of charades or going out with friends to a comedy club. Therapeutic Humor can also be used in a formal setting. An example of this would be a hospital that has humor carts for patients. What's important to emphasize is that Therapeutic Humor can be anything that amuses you and leads you towards better mental and physical health."

"So it's not about becoming a funnier person?" she asked.

"Not unless that's what you desire," said Dr. Alice. "If someone wants to dress in a clown suit to deliver health care, that's great, but it's not about turning anyone into an entertainment center. That might be stressful and actually defeat the whole purpose."

"Well," she said. "That's a lot of words to describe humor."

"And that's why I have come up with only one word that describes the same thing: Humorize. So instead of saying let's embrace humor and laughter to promote health and wellness and a better appreciation of the absurdities that flourish in life, I can simply say: it's time to be Humorized."

"But is that a word?"

"It is now," said Dr. Alice. "I am hoping it catches on because being Humorized is an important factor for your health and well-being."

"It does sound more appealing than taking fish oil pills."

"Then are you ready to hear more?" asked Dr. Alice.

"Right now?"

"Why not? I have the time and there's so much to talk about. Do you have any idea what humor and laughter can do for your heart or for your immune system?"

"No."

"Do you know The Story of Stress and Disease and How Humor Gives it a Happy Ending?"

"No, but I like happy endings."

"Do you know how to create a Humor Self-Portrait and discover your Laughter IQ?"

"No."

"Have you ever gotten together with others to Laugh for the Joy of It?"

"Definitely not."

"Have you ever heard of Coping Humor and how it can reduce the stress in your life?"

"Maybe."

"Do you know how to use the Weapons of Laugh Instruction to add more humor to your life?"

"I never carry any weapons."

"Then there's a lot of fun and facts waiting for you, if you have the time."

She didn't know what to answer. She didn't exactly have plans for the day in case she had to wait hours to see the doctor. However, she wasn't in the mood for a lecture. But how to tactfully say that?

"You may have the time," she finally said. "But I don't know if you have the right audience. I was quite renowned in college for my ability to snore through any lecture."

"Who's talking about lecturing?"

"Aren't you?"

"Me? Lecture? That's not my style. Besides, that wouldn't be fun for you or me, would it?"

"Then what will we do?"

"Chat, play games and share funny stories. I have even been known to panto-mime. So, do you want to begin?"

She agreed even though she still wasn't sure where all this talk about humor was heading. But why not go along for the ride? Wait. Maybe it's time to start saying: Why not go along for the laugh?

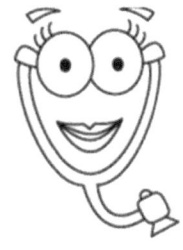

2. Activate Your Humor Antennae and Tune in Humorvision

"I think I'll begin with a pantomime," said Dr. Alice.

"A pantomime?"

But Dr. Alice didn't answer her. Instead, she put a hand on each side of her head with only the index fingers pointing up. She then began wiggling her index fingers asking, "Can you guess what I am doing?"

"I doubt it," she said, shaking her head. "Charades have never been my thing."

"Come on, give it a try. What do my hands remind you of?"

She wanted to say that they reminded her of hands, but she didn't want to disappoint Dr. Alice who looked so, so … enthusiastic? Were her hands some kind of horns? Was the doctor trying to mimic a famous reindeer? This seemed off the wall, but then again, this doctor was so off the wall she might even be from another planet. Another planet? That's it! She said: "You're an alien and those are your antennae!"

"Almost!" Dr. Alice said putting her hands down. "I'm not an alien, at least I don't think so, but I am positioning my Humor Antennae. It's the first thing to do if you want to be Humorized. You need to get these suckers up and activated."

"And are you getting any signals?" she asked.

"Of course. I get them all the time even with my hands at my sides. So if you feel silly acting this out, you don't have to do it."

"That's a relief," she said.

"Where you put your hands doesn't matter. What does matter is becoming more aware of how much humor there is in everyday life even when you least expect it. You need to be primed and ready to enjoy all the absurdities that come your way. That's why you need to activate your Humor Antennae and tune in Humorvision.

"Are you telling me that you find a lot of humor in our overstressed world?" she asked.

"I do," said Dr. Alice. "I've even written and published many of the true and hilarious moments that have come my way in a book called *Where Can I Be Decaffeinated?* I know most of them by heart. Would you like to hear one? It took place quite a while ago but it's still one of my favorites."

"Sure."

*   *   *   *

"Boogie," said my husband, using my nickname, "let's get away this winter."

"You want to get away? Like away, away, as in take a vacation?" I had to make sure that I was hearing what I thought I was hearing.

"Why the surprise?" he asked.

"Maybe, just maybe, it's because the last time we 'vacationed' with the kids it wasn't exactly a dream getaway," I said.

If a vacation is defined as *a period of rest and relaxation*, due to two moments of *unrest and procreation,* I was guaranteed that R 'n' R would elude me for many, many years. Instead, I could look forward to experiencing the definitive oxymoron of the 20th century: the family vacation.

"But the kids are older now," said my husband.

"Older? They are eighteen months and three and a half! And I don't want another experience like the last one." I clearly remember how naive I was to think that a vacation with an infant and a toddler would pose no big problems. I had actually looked forward to having quality time with them. In this state of delusion, I booked a room at a hotel that offered an array of relaxing delights. Unfortunately, I can't tell you what they were since I never got a chance to try any. In fact, I don't remember anything that occurred at the resort except that the room service bill was so high that the hotel manager called to remind us that only a limited number of people were allowed in each room and that the hotel was a family resort with moral standards. I was too inhibited to tell him that the closest I had come to a sexual encounter was startling a fellow guest who obviously thought at five in the morning he could safely retrieve his morning paper in the nude.

"We won't go to a fancy hotel this time," said my husband. "Do you have any other ideas?"

In a perfect world I knew exactly where I would go: Alaska. Now I realize that December in Alaska may not be everyone's idea of an ideal holiday, but I have always dreamed of attending the Bald Eagle Festival that is held every year in the town of Chilkat. I often look at the brochure that says something like this:

Come experience the Alaska Bald Eagle Festival that attracts hordes of doomed salmon, ravenous eagles and half-witted birders who come from all over the world to view this spectacle in the fresh, glacial air. During the day enjoy the thrills and chills of watching hundreds of America's National Bird gorge themselves on salmon that swim up the river to copulate, lay eggs and die. For those guests not hospitalized for hypothermia at the end of the day, the evenings will feature seminars on such provocative subjects like "Why Aren't Bald Eagles Bald?"

However, bringing small children to this event is discouraged for a good reason. Hundreds of hungry grizzly bears also feast on the dying salmon, making it absolutely essential to remain a safe distance away from this spectacle. The festival doesn't want to give a new meaning to the National Park motto: *Take Only Photos, Leave Only Footprints.*

"Boogie, why aren't you answering me?" asked my husband. The sound of his voice woke me from my reverie and reluctantly, I let go of my dreams of eagles, grizzlies and dead fish.

"What were you saying?" I asked.

"I was suggesting that we go to Hawaii."

"Well, why not," I thought, "it will be warm, casual and kid friendly.

Planning the trip was relatively easy. My husband and I agreed that we would only go to one island and stay in a condo for two weeks. While friends exclaimed at the luxurious length of our trip, I knew that I would need two weeks of recovery time before facing the flight home. I also decided that the amenities the condo offered, a washer and a dryer, were more important than water slides and swimming with dolphins.

I was more concerned about being cooped up in a plane with an infant and a toddler. That's why I was delighted to hear upon reaching the gate that a computer glitch had changed our seat assignments and we were now seated separately.

"You mean none of us are together?" I asked.

"That's right," she said.

That was the best news I had heard for a long time. "That's great," I said. "I had no idea that airline policy allowed a toddler to fly without parental supervision, but it works for me. I'm not complaining."

"How old is your child?" asked the employee.

"Three." Maybe I should've kept my mouth shut since magically we were all together again. Oh well, at least I had a moment of bliss.

We didn't have to wait long to board. The agent taking our boarding passes smiled at us and said, "I see that the whole family is taking a vacation."

"Not a vacation," I corrected her. "A vacation is relaxing. We're taking a trip. There's a big difference."

We found our seats and began taking turns either holding our daughter or reading the same books over and over again and coloring at least a hundred pictures. I was having so much fun that it only felt like we had been sitting there for ten days, not two hours, when my son said:

"I need to go pee pee."

I was ready for a break, so I offered to take him. We walked up the aisle to the lavatories in the center of the plane. There was no line, but the sign read *occupied*. My son passed the time by asking me eight times when we would get to Hawaii. I was really relieved when a door finally opened and a man came out accompanied by the loud whoosh of the toilet flushing. I felt my son's hand tighten in mine.

"What's that noise?" he asked.

"Just the toilet flushing."

"That's the toilet?" he asked, backing away from the door. "I am not going in there."

"But sweetie," I said, "It's just that it's a louder noise than usual. It's not going to hurt you."

"I am not going in there," he declared. "That toilet sounds like it's going to suck me out of the plane. Then I would be deaded."

"It's not going to suck you out. I promise."

He wasn't about to buy that. "How do you know?"

"Because I do."

"I am not going in there." I tried every reason, bribe and threat that I could think of to get him into that lavatory. When all that failed, I tried to bodily carry him in, but that didn't work either. He started screaming.

"It's going to suck me out and make me deaded! Help! Help!" I put him down only to hear him moan, "Mommy, I have to go pee pee now!"

What to do? I had no diapers that would fit him since he had been potty trained for months. Luckily at that moment I looked up and saw a man holding a plastic soda cup. Inspiration seized me. I ran back to my seat, grabbed my empty cup while yelling at my husband, "He won't pee in the toilet!" I then rushed back to my son and right there in front of the lavatory door I pulled down his pants, held out the cup and cried, "Go!"

The immediate relief that both he and I felt quickly ended when I realized his cup was going to runneth over. I looked around for help and saw only the fascinated faces of our captive audience. I hoped that a flight attendant would appear but there was not a one in sight. This didn't surprise me. Anyone who has traveled with children knows that flight attendants are so named because as soon as they sense a problem, they take flight. With absolutely no idea what to do, I could only stand there waiting for the lake to become a waterfall while silently cursing the dinky cups the airlines use. Is there some great airplane deity that mandates the use of cups that require ten refills in order to empty a can of soda? However, before the worst could happen, I saw a truly astounding sight: a knight dashing up the aisle to rescue us. Witnesses of this event may state that it was only my husband, yet to this day I swear that I beheld a gallant rescuer of "toddlers in distress" charge forward, holding his daughter in one hand and an empty cup in the other.

"Ready, switch!" he yelled, and miraculously with our son still urinating, we managed to swap cups without spilling a drop. I was so amazed by our sleight of hand that it took me a minute to realize that the noise ricocheting through the plane was the applause from our fellow passengers. Hey, who needs show girls and white tigers when you have a three year old with a full bladder and two plastic cups?

By the time my son was once again clothed he was quite a celebrity, receiving rave reviews that ranged from, "Now that's what I call in-flight entertainment," to "Your son is the ultimate Whiz Kid." Then there is always the person who needs to find the moral in every story. In our case it was the passenger who said, "You really demonstrated the importance of the two parent family."

A few hours later the plane touched down to the sound of the Whiz Kid shouting, "We made it!" His adoring audience applauded once again.

After that, how exciting could the rest of the trip be? It was nice to be away from it all in a condo that overlooked a gorgeous bay framed by a lovely beach … that we rarely visited. All my daughter did was eat the beach while my son refused to even walk on the sand. He would stubbornly stand in a grassy area yards away from the seashore and refuse to move. He was convinced that the bay was like a giant airplane toilet ready to "suck him out and make him deaded." No type of beverage cup could make him change his mind.

*   *   *   *

"I wish I could've seen that," she said.
"It is too bad I can't restage it and charge admission," said Dr. Alice.

"People might pay to see something that funny," she said. "In fact, it's so blatantly funny did you really need to activate your Humor Antennae?"

"Absolutely," said Dr. Alice, "because activating my antennae gave me the Humorvision version. Having my child pee on the floor in front of a bunch of strangers could've been stressful, but by choosing to see the humor in it, I not only amused myself I gave my fellow travelers the chance to laugh with me. How else can you explain a group of strangers coming together to applaud a urinating toddler?"

"I'm not sure if I've ever thought there could be a choice between stress and humor," she said.

"More often than you think, there is a choice. Many funny moments pass us by because we choose to stress over them and not see their lighter side. That's why I came up with the term 'activating your Humor Antennae.' I want people to enthusiastically look for the amusing side of everyday life. And so many hilarious moments exist. Humorvision has unlimited channels and unlimited categories. It might be one of the world's largest satellite dishes. However, funny moments can occur by just turning on one channel, too. Take traveling, for example. As soon as I tune in to one humorous travel story, it makes me think of others. It's a domino humor effect."

"So tuning in to one funny travel story makes you think of others?" she asked.

"It sure does. Every time I think about 'The Whiz Kid' another restroom challenged travel moment always pops up."

"Was this one about your son, too?" she asked.

"No, it's about me."

"You?"

"Yes, I had a 'problem' during a trip to Austria with my daughter."

"Did it happen on an airplane?" she asked.

"No, but I always start the story on the airplane to Vienna where I was seated next to an Englishman who appeared enthused about our destination."

*   *   *   *

"Austria, such a lovely place," he said, "and so much history."

"Really?" I asked.

"Well, of course," he answered, "how else can you describe what was the center of the Holy Roman Empire for hundreds of years?"

I didn't answer him right away because I was confused. Haven't Romans always lived in Rome? And why did he add the word "Holy" to the Roman

Empire? Obviously he did not know what he was talking about so I decided to help him out.

"The Roman Empire was a fascinating time," I said. "Caesar and Antony were a couple of characters, weren't they?"

"I meant the Holy Roman Empire. You know, the center of Christianity for hundreds of years."

Uh oh, he did know what he was talking about. Not wanting to sound stupid I ran the words Austria, Christianity and The Holy Roman Empire through my mind and finally came up with: "That was kind of a Catholic thing, wasn't it?"

Fortunately, he was already moving on to another subject. "Are you planning to visit Schonbrunn Palace?"

"What's that?" I asked.

"You haven't heard of Schonbrunn?" he asked, sounding shocked. "The only palace in Europe that rivals Versailles? The summer home of the Royal Hapsburg family who ruled Austria for centuries?"

"The Hapsburgs? I think I have heard of them, but I can't remember where."

"Do you mind if I ask you why you are going to Austria?" he asked. "Obviously, Austrian history is not your thing. Perhaps you are a hiker, planning to scale the Alps?"

I laughed at that. "Me? Climb mountains? No way. But I am going to Austria for a specific reason."

"Ahh, you are going for the music, Mozart, maybe take in an opera?"

"No, no. I am going there to eat pastries."

"To eat pastries?" he repeated.

"I always watch this television show called *Great Chefs of the World*. Last year, they had a whole series of programs on Austrian cuisine. I was amazed to find out that Austrian desserts are in a class of their own."

"Are you serious?" he asked. "Are you really going all the way to Vienna to eat cake?"

"I plan to do a lot more than eat cake. There are also tortes, strudels, and creme schnittes. Austria is one of the great 'sweet tooth experiences' in the world."

"Can't you get dessert in The Colonies?"

"Not like you can in Vienna. The famous Austrian chef, Wolfgang Puck, who now resides in The Colonies once said: 'A pastry in Austria is not a dessert. It is a way of life.'"

"I still can't believe that you know about creme schnittes but not the Hapsburgs."

"Oh, I just remembered that I have heard of the Hapsburgs," I said excitedly. "I did research on the most famous pastry shops in Vienna and I came across one called the Cafe Demel that claimed that they made pastries for the Hapsburgs."

"I'm sure that you must have heard of at least one Hapsburg, Marie Antoinette."

"Marie Antoinette was from Austria?"

"Yes, she was a Hapsburg, an Austrian princess born and raised there before she married the French King."

"Then that explains it!"

"Explains what?" asked my companion.

"If she was from Austria, is it any wonder that she said: 'Let them eat cake!'"

The plane landed soon after that revelation and my journey began. I started tasting my way through Vienna, Innsbruck and Salzburg. Okay, so I did more than taste. I gorged on creme shnittes, mocha krapfes, doboshtortes, truffeltortes, kaffetortes, mohntortes and sachertortes. Yet one dessert still eluded me: the famous Zaunerstollen.

There was a reason for this. Zauner's Konditorrei, considered by many to be Austrian's finest, is located in Bad Ischl, a small town located in the center of the beautiful Lake District renowned for its hot springs. However, being in the middle of nowhere was not going to stop me from sampling a Zaunerstollen when all we had to do was rent a car in Salzburg and drive about 75 miles. Unfortunately, upon arrival I realized that I had forgotten the guidebook with the bakery's address. Since Bad Ischl was a good-sized town, achieving my culinary goal was not going to be easy as I thought. I drove and drove, but no Zauner's. Finally, tired from all the driving around, I decided it was time for a rest.

My daughter and I found a lovely esplanade, a park by a river, so I pulled in, parked the car and suggested that we make a picnic out of the rolls and cheese that we had brought. It was a beautiful spot, nestled next to a turquoise river. A charming pedestrian bridge connected the park to the picturesque town on the other side. We sat down on a shady bench and began eating. However, within minutes, I discovered a problem with the park. It lacked restrooms and I was suddenly feeling that strong urge one often feels when traveling.

"Hey," I said getting up. "I have to go."

"Now, Mom? Can't you wait until I've finished?"

"No! I really gotta go!" I said, taking off and hauling my butt across the pedestrian bridge towards an outdoor cafe brightened with red and white umbrellas that would have what I urgently needed.

"At least wait for me!" she yelled as she scrambled across the bridge after me.

"I can't wait! I may not make it!" was my answer, as I accelerated my pace towards the cafe where I ran in the door and headed straight for the bathroom. Some time later I walked out of the restroom to find my daughter with a look of pure bliss fastened on her face.

"Look!" she said, pointing to the floor where the word *Zauners* was written in bold, gold letters. I then turned to my right and couldn't believe what I had missed: several huge glass cases glimmering with the most incredible array of desserts I have ever seen. I said a silent prayer of thanks before settling down to eat a pastry, so delectable, so rich and so flavorful that I still think of it as Zaunerlicious.

✳   ✳   ✳   ✳

"That's not only funny," she said, "it's a story I can relate to."

"You also have a sweet tooth?"

"I do," she said.

"My own personal motto could be *Let Me Eat Cake*," said Dr. Alice. "Sometimes I wish I could start a pastry revolution! However, I just can't find any data to support the need for more sweets in our life. I'll just stick to my Humor Revolution because unlike sachertortes, humor benefits the mind, heart, lungs, and immune system. It also reduces the release of stress hormones while increasing flexibility, creativity and energy levels."

"That's a lot of claims," she said.

"Yes, but they're all true."

"Like?"

"I don't want to just fire off facts," said Dr. Alice. "I've already been warned that lecturing might put you to sleep."

"That's true," she said.

"So why don't we play a game instead?"

"Is it called *Doctor*?" she asked.

"No, it's not," said Dr. Alice laughing. "The game I want to play is called *Laugh for Your Life*. It's a lot like the television game show *Who Wants To Be A Millionaire*? Do you remember that?"

"Of course."

"Even if you weren't, it's easy to play. I'm the host with a list of questions about health and humor. As the contestant, you get to try and answer them."

"And if I get all the right answers, do I win a million dollars?"

"No, but you might win a million laughs," said Dr. Alice, before asking the first question.

Gelotology is a field of science that studies:
A. The effects of gelato on the ice cream receptors in the brain
B. How the overproduction of gelatin is causing global warming
C. Humor and laughter and how they affect the human body

"So, what do you think?" asked Dr. Alice.

"What am I supposed to think, Dr. Alice? You just asked me about ice cream receptors, gelatin and global warming. What have they got to with humor and health?"

"Everything."

"Now I'm really confused," she said.

"That's because you haven't given yourself Permission to Play."

"Permission to Play?"

"Being Humorized is more than activating antennae to enjoy the absurdities in everyday life," said Dr. Alice. "You also need to give yourself Permission to Play."

"With what?"

"With whatever you find. That's what I am doing with these questions. I could make them all serious but isn't it more fun this way?"

"It is," she said. "I just wasn't expecting it."

"Of course you weren't because you are an adult and in our society adults rarely play, right?"

"I have to say," she said, "that I rarely think about playing."

"Not many adults do which is why I want you to consider this. If a young child sees a puddle what does he or she usually do?"

"Jump in it!"

"Exactly, but if you see a puddle, do you usually jump in it?" asked Dr. Alice.

"No!"

"In fact, you might say: 'Oh my gosh, it's a puddle. I don't want to jump in it because I might get my pants wet and my shoes muddy. Even worse, I might slip and fall and break my leg ... and then I'll have to go to a hospital ... and have surgery ... and miss work ... and not be able to pay the mortgage on my house ... and then I'll lose everything and my life will be ruined....'"

She cracked up as Dr. Alice said: "Hey, I might be exaggerating but what I described is not that far off. And guess what? Ceasing to play is not a healthy way to live because our bodies thrive on joy and fun. An unknown person said it so well: *We stop playing as we age and we age because we stop playing.*"

"So I need to give myself Permission to Play?"

"Yes. And it isn't that hard," said Dr. Alice. "I'm not asking you to jump in any puddles. All I'm asking you to do is play with a few questions. So, why not just relax and enjoy being Humorized."

"That's certainly a novel thought."

"But novelty can be so much fun," said Dr. Alice. "Now, do you need me to repeat the question?"

"No. The obvious and final answer is C."

"Gelotology is the field of science devoted to studying the effects of humor and laughter on health. The word itself comes from the Greek word, gelos, which can mean laugh, laughter or laughing."

"Who came up with that word?" she asked.

"Most people credit Dr. William Fry, Jr., a Professor Emeritus of Psychiatry at Stanford University who began his research into humor and health in the sixties and came up with a startling answer to this question:

Laughter has similar physical benefits to:
A. Eating Fiberlicious
B. Sniffing Fish Oils
C. Keeping a pair of jogging shoes in the closet
D. Exercising

"Dr. Alice, that card can't possibly say that!"

"It doesn't, but didn't you find it amusing?"

"I did."

"And your answer?"

"D," she said. "Laughter is like exercise and that's final."

"And do you find that surprising?"

"I do," she said. "I had no idea."

"It surprised Dr. Fry, too, because he thought laughter might have a negative physical effect on the body. Imagine his surprise and relief when he discovered that no one actually dies laughing."

"Does this mean that if I lie on my couch watching a funny DVD and laughing, my body receives the same benefits as if I were working out?"

"Wouldn't that be nice," said Dr. Alice. "We could call this *The Couch Potato Work Out*. And laughter does have the same physical benefits as exercise.[3] Both can cause an initial increase in heart rate and blood pressure, but that is quickly followed by a decrease in heart rate and blood pressure that is beneficial. Exercise and laughter also increase ventilation in the lungs, another benefit to the body. But while laughing 100 times is like 15 minutes on an exercise bike,[4] it's not easy to quantify or sustain hearty laughter, is it? We usually laugh in shorter bursts, so I would not call laughter a substitute for exercise. But the physical effects are only part of the picture. Like exercise, smiling and laughing feel wonderful and I'm not just speaking of a fleeting feeling. Dr. Fry himself said it so well: *I believe humor is both a contributor and a manifestation of our mental health. It reflects a positive orientation to life and a sense of wellbeing. Humor is not just a maneuver or a joke. It gives us a broader, deeper view of life. It influences the relationships between human beings, as well as their relationship to the world."*

"That's lovely," she said.

"And we've only just begun," said Dr. Alice. "Research has shown that humor and laughter cause so many positive effects to the mind and body, it's like having a total internal body massage. However, before we go any further I need to make a crucial point: only one type of laughter causes these positive effects."

"There's always a catch," she said.

"Yes, but this one's easy to grasp."

Only type of laughter produces beneficial health effects.:
A. Laughter-Lite
B. Laughy Laughter
C. Mirthful Laughter

"The answer is B, Laughy Laughter," she said.

"And is that your final answer?"

"No, I just wanted to say Laughy Laughter. My final answer is C, Mirthful Laughter."

"Which is correct," said Dr. Alice," because Mirthful Laughter is the foundation of Therapeutic Humor. It's important to understand that we laugh for more than one reason: because we're nervous, embarrassed or feel awkward. But only Mirthful Laughter causes the cascade of positive effects to our mind and bodies.[5] For that to happen, you need to have a warm-hearted experience that leaves you feeling optimistic and relaxed. However, it is very important to point out that you don't have to laugh out loud to for this to happen. Mirthful Humor works just as well. What's important is having the mirthful experience which needs to feel comfortable, comforting and safe."

"Safe?"

"Yes, Mirthful Laughter or Humor never hurts anyone's feelings. It may make fun of people's behaviors and idiosyncrasies, but it never puts anyone down or makes fun of whom they are. In the airplane story with my son, I just have fun with his behavior. When he is yelling that the toilet is going to suck him out and make him deaded, I don't respond by putting him down and calling him a loser because he won't pee in the airplane john."

"That's actually a pretty funny thought," she said with a smile.

"I'm not saying put down humor can't be funny and it's certainly not my job or place to tell anyone not to use it. People should be free to enjoy whatever humor appeals to them. I call this The First Amendment of Humor."

"A Constitutional right?"

"Absolutely," said Dr. Alice. "However, if you want to gain health benefits from humor, you have to experience Mirthful Laughter or Humor which can reduce tension not create it. It can forge bonds between people, not divide them. It's empowering and allows us to see new possibilities. Someone, and I wish I knew who once said it so well: *Mirthful Laughter may point out the weaknesses of Humanity but it does not contain contempt nor does it leave a sting. In fact, it may even offer hope.*"

"Hope?"

"Yes, there have been studies that show that humor can increase hope." [6]

"That's a rather moving thought, Dr. Alice."

"I think so."

"Yet it also makes me think of something rather funny," she said.

"What?"

"Mirthful Laughter makes me think of *Star Wars*."

"*Star Wars*?" asked Dr. Alice.

"Yes! Do you remember how *The Force* is the power that fuels the good guys in *Star Wars*?"

"Of course!"

"Isn't Mirthful Laughter *The Force* in the world of Therapeutic Humor?"

"It is," said Dr. Alice. "What a great thought except ..."

"Except?"

"Perhaps we ought to say it's *The Laugh* in the world of Therapeutic Humor. Or better yet, *May The Laugh Be With You*."

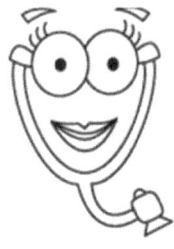

Laughing with Dr. Alice
Experience the Power of Joy

3. *Laugh for Your Life*

"I hope you want to keep playing *Laugh for Your Life*," said Dr. Alice. "I still have exciting info to share about humor, ice cream and global warming."

"I'd like to hear more, but not about ice cream and global warming, Dr. Alice."

"Okay, then how about seeing what humor can do for one end of your body."

Mirthful Laughter has been shown to:
A. Improve your feet by experiencing Hoof and Laugh Syndrome
B. Increase creativity and the ability to solve problems

"Hoof and Laugh Syndrome? Dr. Alice, how do think this stuff up?"

"I just give my mind Permission to Play, and I have such fun with it. I wish I had a racehorse so I could name him that. Wouldn't it be great to hear an announcer say: 'Hoof and Laugh just won the Kentucky Derby.'"

"Well, I hope you get your racehorse someday, but that's not my answer. I doubt gelotologists study humor and feet so my final answer is B."

"Increasing creativity and the ability to solve problems," said Dr. Alice.

"My mind does feel clear and refreshed after a good laugh," she said.

"And that might have to do with joy and laughter causing the release of endorphins from the brain," [7] said Dr. Alice. "Endorphins are referred to as the feel good hormones because they are natural opium-like substances that may explain why people experience less pain when Humorized.[8,9] However, there is another reason why humor may have such a powerful effect on the mind. It's a well-known fact that most emotions light up only one small part of the brain, but not humor! Your entire brain can light up when you laugh!"

"What do you mean by light up?" she asked.

"When people are exposed to different emotional triggers like anger or humor, scientists can scan their brains to see what areas become active or light up. They've found that humor and laughter start on the left side of the brain and then quickly move to include the right side.[10,11] This may explain why a smile or a chuckle enhances communication, creativity, problem solving and enables you to think more clearly."

"So people have studied this?"

"Yes," said Dr. Alice. "A couple of studies showed that the formal use of humor improved the outcome of serious work, creativity, problem solving and communication.[12,13] Another study exposed half of a group to a humorous experience before giving the whole group a tricky problem to solve.[14] Guess who solved the problem better?"

"The group with Hoof and Laugh Syndrome?"

Dr. Alice smiled. "I don't think so. The group exposed to humor solved the problem better which suggests that humor may make the mind more flexible and receptive. That's why I use humor to teach humor."

"Your own method of hands-on learning?"

"I prefer to call it Laughs-on Learning," said Dr. Alice. "You're smiling again. That means your mind is primed and ready to find out more about humor and health."

What common activity appears to prevent heart disease?
A. Brushing your teeth
B. Chatting on the phone
C. Brushing your teeth while chatting on the phone
D. Experiencing hearty laughter while watching a comedy show

"The answer is obvious," she said.

"That chatting on the phone prevents heart disease?" asked Dr. Alice.

"If that were true there would be no heart disease," she said. "My final answer is D, but what I also want to know is this. Who thought of studying the effect of humor on the heart? That in and of itself is fascinating."

"It is a fascinating story that begins on a remote tropical island in the South Pacific. Johnny Depp, now a highly-respected pirate gelotologist, was relaxing on a white sand beach, surrounded by half-clad Polynesian beauties plying him with native delicacies when suddenly a profound question about heart disease and humor effervesced from deep within him just like the bubbles foaming from his tropical drink."

"Dr. Alice?"

"Yes?"

"I hate to break the tropical mood, but I think I'd prefer the true version."

"Okay, I'll leave Johnny, the beautiful island and the half-clad Polynesian beauties," said Dr. Alice. "Instead, I'll start by saying that it's an accepted fact that exercise benefits the heart, right?"

"Right!"

"We also know that exercise and laughter have similar physical effects on the body. So, doesn't it make sense to ask, if exercise is good for the heart, then shouldn't laughter be beneficial also?"

"That does make sense," she said.

"A team of researchers that included Dr. Lee Berk, a scientist with numerous publications on humor and health, decided to study this.[15] 48 patients who had recently recovered from a heart attack were divided into two groups of 24 each. Both groups received standard cardiac rehabilitation which included medications and counseling about Lifestyle Choices for a healthier heart like diet, exercise and ceasing to smoke."

She visibly shuddered at those words. "I think Lifestyle Challenges is a better term. Eating a bowl of *Fiberlicous* or working out on *The Rack* is not easy or fun."

"Lifestyle Choices aren't always easy," said Dr. Alice, "but they are known to contribute to heart health and were recommended to both groups. However, a new Lifestyle Choice was added to the second group. And this one was anything but challenging! All they had to do was enjoy a 20 to 30 minute humorous show of their choice on a daily basis. At the end of a year a second heart attack occurred in 42% of the people who had not watched a funny show on a daily basis."

"That's a huge number," she said.

"It is. What else do you think they found?"

"Well," she said, "I know it wasn't anything about brushing your teeth."

"They found that the group who had been Humorized required less medication and, more significantly, only 8% had a second heart attack. This is an extremely significant difference, 8% versus 42%. In fact, it's downright astonishing and once again brings up the important point I made earlier: How you live your life contributes so much to how long your life will be. And humor may play a major role."

"That is something," she said. "I wonder why this study didn't make more of a splash in the news."

"As I've said before, medicine is a business and there's nothing to be gained financially from humor. If someone had come up with a drug that could do this, he would be able to buy a remote tropical island. But money isn't the whole story. I also think that despite all the evidence to support it, the importance of humor as a lifestyle, is still not taken seriously. Maybe we need to start offering a Nobel Humor Prize. Isn't that a great idea? Imagine, inspiring brilliant people to come up with the best way to fill the world with laughter."

"While I hate to sound pessimistic, I don't think that will ever happen," she said.

"Probably not," said Dr. Alice, "but at least some other research supported this finding. Another study showed that there appears to be an inverse relationship between heart disease and humor.[16] That means the more you laugh, the less likely you are to get heart disease."

"And do we know why laughter appears to help prevent heart disease?"

"We are figuring this out," said Dr. Alice. "One intriguing possibility was discovered by Dr. Steve Miller, a cardiologist and Director of Preventive Cardiology at the University of Maryland." [17]

"And did he discover this on some remote Greek island surrounded by the glistening blue of the Mediterranean and enticing dark-eyed beauties?" she asked.

"Sadly for Dr. Miller, I'm pretty sure he was stuck in Baltimore when he decided to find out if humor could increase blood flow in our arteries. Do you know why this is important?"

"I think so," she said, "but run it by me again anyway."

"Organs in general do better when the arteries that supply them with blood are relaxed and open because extra blood means extra nourishment. The opposite is also true. If an organ, like the heart, doesn't get enough blood because an artery is too narrow or constricted, this can cause damage and even a heart attack. Got that?"

"Got it!" she said.

"So Dr. Miller asked, can humor also dilate vessels and offer organs like the heart protection from disease? To answer this he studied and compared two groups. The first watched a funny video while the second viewed a film considered to be mentally stressful. Images of arteries were monitored in both groups and guess what he found?"

"That humor will dilate blood vessels?"

"It sure does," said Dr. Alice. "In the Humorized group, arteries dilated up to 22%, while the blood vessels of those being exposed to the stress movies narrowed up to 35%. This effect lasted 45 minutes.[17] It appears that humor and laughter may play an important role in keeping arteries open and the heart healthy."

"Does that mean it's okay to start scarfing down double cheeseburgers as long as you laugh?" she asked.

"Now you're dreaming," said Dr. Alice, "because at this point humor is not a substitute for other heart healthy Lifestyle Choices. It's an addition, but at least it's a fun and entertaining one."

"May I ask one more question?"

"Ask as many as you like," said Dr. Alice.

"Does this mean that if I have a heart attack, I should try to think of something funny while I wait for the paramedics?"

"While I like the idea I somehow don't see anyone with crushing chest pain being able to think about their favorite joke or Seinfeld episode. The focus of these findings needs to be on preventing heart disease in healthy people or in trying to avert a second major heart event in those with previous problems."

"Oh well," she said. "It's still pretty amazing to think that there are hard core facts showing how humor protects the heart."

"There certainly are, but perhaps we should call them heart core facts. And that's not even all that humor and laughter can do."

What increases the ability of certain immune cells to fight cancer?
A. Drinking a daily martini laced with Viagra
B. Eating cinnamon coated soybeans soaked in green tea
C. Taking time to enjoy the absurdities in life

"I wish the answer was A," she said. "If I could come up with a cocktail that enhances sex and fights cancer, I might make enough money to make Bill Gates look needy."

"Maybe you should look into this," said Dr. Alice.

"But not until you've explained the real answer which is C, that enjoying humor increases the ability of cells that fight cancer. This is so specific and, and ..."

"Surprising?" asked Dr. Alice.

"More than surprising. I am totally ..."

"Gobsmacked?"

"Gob what?" she asked.

"Gobsmacked. It's a British word for more than amazed."

"Then I am gobsmacked."

"But the facts are in," said Dr. Alice. "Our immune system is made up of many different types of cells that have specific functions or jobs. Studies have shown that humor and laughter can increase the quantity and the ability of these cells to function.[18,19,20] In one study, blood samples were taken from a group of people who watched a funny video of their choice and from a similar group unexposed to a humorous experience. They found that the blood from the Humorized group had a significant increase in the activity of immune cells, called natural killer cells, when compared to the other group. Natural killer cells are very important because they are specifically active against cancer."[20]

"Are you saying that humor increases the ability of a killer cell to kill?"

"Yes I am and wouldn't that make a great horror movie? I can picture it now. A dinghy room with a natural killer cell lounging on a tattered couch while it watches reruns of *I Love Lucy*. The cell starts laughing and suddenly it has more ability to kill …"

"Dr. Alice?"

"Yes?"

"Maybe you should just stick with your Humor Revolution and answering a question I have. Were these subjects cancer patients?"

"No," said Dr. Alice, "and that's an important point. These studies looked at how immune cells from healthy people fight cancer cells in a laboratory setting. So we still don't know how this translates into real life. We don't have the evidence to say that humor may prevent cancer or prolong life in cancer patients. Happily, there is one thing I can say without any reservations. Laughter does not cause your hair to fall out."

She smiled. "I'll buy that."

"And while humor and laughter are still not accepted treatments for cancer," said Dr. Alice, "they may give cancer patients a leg up.[19,21] Adding giggles and guffaws can also give a tremendous boost to the quality of life as well as being an easy and enjoyable option to add to other modalities."

"I've heard about cancer support groups that use humor," she said, "but it never occurred to me that they were doing anything but boosting the patients' moods while offering emotional support."

"And right now, we can't say any more than that," said Dr. Alice. "However, since humor does effect and enhance the immune system, I think it's important to encourage anyone with cancer or any other ongoing disease to seek out support groups that use smiles and laughter."

"It certainly won't hurt anyone," she said.

"No," said Dr. Alice. "And it's not just cancer patients that need to be smiling and laughing more. Natural killer cells are also active against many common viruses as well."

"So humor may help the immune system with life-threatening diseases and common illnesses?"

"Yes, in fact it's now time to find out if humor can help with the most common disease of all."

Being Humorized can increase antibodies that fight:
A. The common cold
B. The uncommon cold
C. The bitter cold of winter in Los Angeles

"The answer is *A*," she said, "but antibodies are ..."

"They are proteins also known as immunoglobulins. They are produced by the immune system in response to the presence of bacteria or viruses in the body. You have an antibody in your saliva called immunoglobulin A that helps ward off the common cold and when you are Humorized it has been shown to increase." [22,23]

"So if I'm exposed to a cold, I should start watching funny videos?"

"It can't hurt," said Dr. Alice, "and you will also be boosting many other parts of your immune system as well."

"It's pretty mind-boggling to think of all the ways humor effects the immune system."

"And I haven't even mentioned so many of them like what humor does for cytokines, interferons, granulocytes, etc., but I think that's enough terms for now. I don't want to send you out of here screaming with your hair on end."

"Good idea," she said.

"However, I do want to mention one more easily understood point. The benefits to the immune system are not just a quick fix. Just 20 to 30 minutes a day of humor and laughter can have an effect that can last up to 12 hours and possibly longer." [7,20]

"That's impressive."

"It is when you think how little time 20 to 30 minutes a day is. That's quite a reward for your body."

"It is, but ..."

"But?"

"Even though you refer to humor as The Feel Good Lifestyle, isn't it also another Lifestyle Challenge? That may not be a lot of time, but it's still something that I'll have to actively think about adding to my life."

"But is it really a challenge?" asked Dr. Alice. "How can encouraging people to take the time to enjoy smiling, giggling or a huge belly laugh for just twenty minutes a day be challenging? I am not asking you to give up any of your favorite foods or get out of bed at six AM to jog on a gloomy morning. The Humor Revolution is simply about setting aside more time to bask in life's enjoyable moments that also happen to enhance your mind and body. This is the ultimate win-win situation. So instead of thinking as humor as a Lifestyle Challenge, why not think of it as a Lifestyle Treat?"

"So I should treat myself to more humor?"

"Why not? There must be a reason why we are the only species with the ability to smile. Why have that capability if it isn't important on a physical and mental level? Even a child born blind and deaf can spontaneously smile and laugh, so it's obviously an innate and vital part of our being."

"I do agree with you, Dr. Alice, and I would like to start setting aside more time to smile and giggle, but so much of the time I'm so busy and stressed out finding extra minutes in the day to laugh might be difficult."

"I completely understand that and I'm glad you brought this up, because it's so important to understand that stress has the opposite effect of humor on the body. Stressing makes your body more vulnerable to disease. When you don't take the time to smile and laugh and instead stress, you are subjecting yourself to a double negative whammy that isn't healthy for you physically or mentally. This is why The Humor Revolution is not just about adding more humor and laughter to your life. It's also about reducing stress. It's a package deal."

"A package deal?"

"Yes, you need to laugh more and stress less for your mind and for your body."

"That makes The Humor Revolution trickier, doesn't it?" she said.

"Yes, but the end result will be worth it because stress has a huge negative impact on our health. Do you know that it's generally accepted that at least 70% of all disease is associated with stress?"

"70%?"

"Yes," said Dr. Alice, "and that's why we need to take some time and try to figure out why we spend so much time stressing."

"And we do," she said. "Like a lot of other people, I am often stressed out."

"Are you?"

"Don't you believe me?" she asked.

"Oh, I believe you," said Dr. Alice. "And I agree that in general we are a pretty stressed out bunch. However, do you truly think life is more stressful than it used to be or have we just reached a point where we actually embrace stress as if it were an old, dear friend?"

"Wait a minute," she said. "Are you suggesting that we're intentionally embracing stress?"

"I am."

"I've never thought of that."

Then maybe it's time you did."

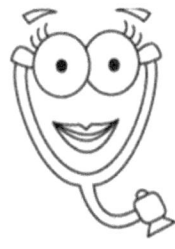

Laughing with Dr. Alice
Experience the Power of Joy

4. Is that a Wooly Mammoth or Am I Just Stressed Out?

"Dr. Alice, I want to make sure that I understand you," she said. "Do you really believe that people today embrace stress?"

"I do."

"I have a hard time with that," she said. "It seems to me that everyone does nothing but complain about it."

"I agree that people constantly talk about stress," said Dr. Alice, "but are they truly complaining?'

"Aren't they?" she asked.

"I wonder about that," said Dr. Alice. "If people dislike stress so much why do so many of us live our lives as if we are over caffeinated and in need of a teddy bear to hug?"

"You've mentioned that funny image before," she said. "People running around clutching teddy bears while their eyes bug out and their hair stands on end."

"And the reason that I've brought it up again is because it's not far from the truth. Carolyn Hax, a columnist for the Washington Post, said the same thing in a different way. She describes us as having … *a societal madness for being 18 people at once … We aren't just parents, we parent. We don't have jobs, we have careers. We don't just enroll our children in an institution, we assume its burdens.*"

"A societal madness? That's a pretty strong statement."

"But it's true because stressing is such a universal phenomenon."

"I won't argue that," she said.

"But why are we living like this? Does it somehow make people feel that their lives are busy and meaningful?"

"You may have a point there," she said. "If I'm not super busy I almost feel like there must be something wrong with me or my life."

"And no one wants to feel like that, do they?"

"No," she said. "You might feel left out."

"And that may explain why everyone is jumping on the 'stressed out bandwagon.'"

"That's an interesting way of putting it."

"It may be interesting, but all this stressing is harmful because it dulls our minds and makes our bodies more susceptible to disease. Stress also prevents us from using humor which energizes our minds and makes our bodies less susceptible to disease."

"That's not good."

"No, it isn't," said Dr. Alice. "That's why it's important to try to figure out why we spend so much time stressing."

"That's okay as long as you don't stress me out over it," she said.

"Don't worry about that. I like to use Laughs on Learning, remember?"

"I do," she said, "and it would be nice to make stress laughable."

"And there can be a choice between stressing and laughing. However nowadays we lean towards stressing. Being 'all stressed out' has become such an accepted part of our daily lives that a traditional greeting has even changed. Not that long ago when people met, they said:

Greeter #1: Hi there, how are you?

Greeter #2: I'm fine, thanks. How are you?"

"Doesn't that still happen?" she asked.

"Not very often," said Dr. Alice. "Nowadays, the conversation is much more likely to go like this:

Greeter #1: How are you?

Greeter #2: I'm all stressed out."

"I do hear that a lot," she admitted.

"Try more than a lot," said Dr. Alice. "My husband comes home from work and when I ask, 'How are you?' he says: 'I'm all stressed out.' I call a friend and ask the same question and what do I hear? 'I'm all stressed out.' The word 'fine' is so rarely used that I think it may be on the endangered word list. In fact, it may soon end up in the great word heaven in the sky."

"A great word heaven in the sky?" she asked. "What's that?"

"I imagine it as a place where discarded words eternally float around listening to soothing music," said Dr. Alice.

She sighed. "That sounds so peaceful and relaxing."

"But you do have a choice here. You can choose to smile and relax more. I grew up in the fifties and sixties and I don't recall people stressing all the time. Why now?"

"Isn't life today just more complicated?" she asked.

"But there are so many more conveniences," said Dr. Alice. "Which makes me wonder, is life really more complicated or are we just making it so? Are we creating Man-made Stress?"

"I don't have the answer."

"I may not either, but I have spent some time thinking about this, particularly in regard to women our age."

"We are a stressed out group," she said. "Work, kids, carpooling, you name it."

"I have named it," said Dr. Alice. "I've called it *More Than A Bad Hair Day*. It's a look at the last part of the 20th century and the start of the new one. And while it may not be the definitive answer as to why the female sex is all stressed out, at least I had a lot fun writing it."

"So it won't stress me out to hear it?"

"I promise that you can listen to this whole piece without needing a teddy bear to hug."

*   *   *   *

More than A Bad hair Day

The Sixties

The seeds of stressing began in a decade better called "The Sexties." The reason: the birth of the Sexual Revolution. Remarkably, this landmark event wasn't led by a general or a comrade, but by a Pill. The Pill I refer to is a tiny tablet that turned the dating game into the mating game. Now, one could fornicate without the fear that what came out of man would, nine months later, come out of woman. This new freedom gave rise to a new term: Casual Sex. This phrase was coined in order to distinguish Casual Sex from Serious Sex, a form of behavior usually found in non-human animals of lesser intelligence. At first glance the emergence of the birth control pill might appear to be a way to decrease stress; however I believe that it actually increased sexual angst. Women, who once might have saved sex for marriage, were suddenly faced with so many men and too few reasons to just say no. This initiated a form of mental perturbation where females would torture themselves with questions like: Should I do it on the first date, the second date or should I wait months? Will it be a relationship or just sex? Am I acting like a loose woman or am I asserting my own sexuality? Frankly, I think that it says a lot for my gender that the sexual revolution didn't make all women sexually insane.

The Seventies

"The Women's Liberation Movement" arrives and suddenly females are told that being a "Stay at Home Mom" is a mind numbing experience. All women should work outside the home, i.e., in the "Real World" in order to achieve emotional and intellectual fulfillment. Thousands of women listened and began marching out of their mundane routines to become part of a second mundane routine. To further inspire us females, bras became a symbol of our oppression and we were encouraged to burn them, preferably, when they were off. However, amidst all this hoopla, one question was never addressed: How did having *two* full-time jobs get defined as "liberation?"

There were a few brave souls who chose not to bring all this stress into their lives. However, they were not given much encouragement. They were instead subjected to comments like: "You mean you just stay at home with your kids?" which sent their stress-o-meters off the wall making "Stay at Home Moms" a rare breed. Some experts predict that this breed may soon become extinct, which is why we need to set aside more than wildlife reserves. Yes, the time has come to create "Domestic Life Reserves" where moms and kids can roam together in peace.

The Eighties

By now the female gender is hoping that this decade will introduce ways to alleviate stress. Forget that. The eighties burst upon the scene with "The War On Cellulite." Now, women are supposed to not only work two full-time jobs, but during all our free time we are also expected to achieve what I call: "The Fit Fountain of Youth Look." To accomplish this, women needed to engage in some form of exercise that makes one pant and sweat, be it jogging, cycling, aerobics, jazzercise, or stepping. Soon, working out became almost as important as working out of the house.

Another option did emerge for females with money: plastic surgery. With a little help from a knife, a needle or a body vacuum, one could be remodeled, reduced, enlarged, sucked or tucked. This cost big bucks, but many were willing to sacrifice certain amenities or go after that third job in order to become society's ideal: a toned toothpick. As tiring or expensive as all this may sound, there was one positive aspect to "The War on Cellulite," the return of the bra. I guess all that bouncing around made people realize the bra is more than just a symbol.

The Nineties

If the eighties could be called "The Fit Fountain of Youth Look," the nineties should be called "The Face Fountain of Youth Look." Females were sent a definite message by the powers that be that any wrinkle or line is a feminine crime. The "good" news is that a national leader emerged to head the new skin patrol unit: Botox. Now, one didn't have to subject herself to the surgeon's knife in order to achieve "The Face Fountain of Youth Look." One's character lines were just a couple of injections away from disappearing, for a few months anyway. The "sad" news is that Botox has eradicated a great American tradition: the Tupperware party. With so many women desperate to have their faces smoothed out by paralyzing their muscles, the Botox party has replaced the gathering where women once ate, chatted and bought rubber-like containers. Now they gather to eat, chat and buy rubber-like faces.

The New Millennium

Stress has become such an essential part of our lives that I believe that if we are not stressing, we often feel left out or worse, unimportant. In other words, if you're not "stressed out over your busy life" something must be wrong with you. To accommodate this 'new life vision' our language has started changing in order to remind us that we should avoid relaxation at all costs. Taking a vacation is now a "Working Vacation" while one doesn't just take a walk anymore. They need to go "Power Walking." What's next? "Power Eating?" "Power Sex?" "A Working Christmas?"

To conclude, being a modern day woman can be a totally stressful experience if we attempt to embrace all the things we are 'supposed' to do: to have a productive career, be a great mom and wife, be toned and fit, and to top it off, avoid aging. It's no wonder that "I'm stressed out" is now the second most common phrase in the English language surpassed only by "I'll have a #3 and can you supersize that?"

*   *   *   *

"That didn't stress me out," she said, "but it wasn't all funny. Parts of *More Than a Bad Hair Day* are almost, well, sad."

"Stress does have a sad side."

"A sad side?"

"Yes, because when you or anyone else starts stressing over this and that all day long, this literally prevents you from experiencing the richness found in many of life's moments. In other words 'stressing' can disconnect you from so much of what life has to offer. This disconnect can lead to a feeling of sadness which may cause even more anxiety. Happiness and pleasure depend on connecting with other people and with the joy that comes from enjoying the present. This point is well illustrated in the story of my son refusing to use the airplane lavatory. By choosing to see the humor, not the stress in the situation I was able to enjoy a rich, amusing and memorable moment that connected me with dozens of strangers."

"I have to say that I have never thought of stress in that light before."

"Maybe you should. I even have a fun way to think about this. Do you remember how we talked about stress narrowing arteries while humor relaxes and opens them?"

"I do," she said.

"Think of stress as narrowing your arteries and narrowing your mind, because as I just pointed out every time you stress you limit your opportunities to savor life and tune in Humorvision. However, when you smile and laugh both your arteries and mind open up."

"That is something for me to think about."

"I hope that it's something that everyone will think about it," said Dr. Alice, "because it's not just women facing Man-made Stress. It's men and children, too. I'm sure many a man could write their version of *More Than a Bad Hair Day*. As for children, I am very concerned for them because too many kids are being raised to think of life as one long class or activity. I recently talked to a parent who proudly listed everything her four-year old twins did in a week: pre-school, soccer, gymnastics, music and me, art and yoga. Talk about pressure."

"Did you say anything?" she asked.

"No, but I wanted to ask if both kids also took Hula. But I didn't because most likely those poor kids would now be wearing grass skirts every week because being busy to the point of stressing out is now the 'in' thing."

"You might be right," she said. "It has become difficult to enjoy 'down time.' I often feel like I always need to be doing something. It's like there must be something wrong with me if I want to spend a weekend relaxing and doing very little."

"I understand," said Dr. Alice. "It's almost like people are afraid of just being or relaxing."

"You may have a point there. Just doing nothing does sound a bit scary."

"But it isn't! It's wonderful. My husband and I have a small cabin in an undeveloped mountain area north of Los Angeles with no lake and no downhill skiing. People always ask: 'What do you do there?'"

"And what do you say?" she asked.

"The truth. We do nothing, except read, rest, walk, look at birds and take the time to be with each other. We are free to spend hours endlessly chatting. This connecting is as much fun to me as swimming or downhill skiing! Yet people often look at me like I'm nuts when I describe how little we do because we live in a society where keeping busy to the point of stress appears to be a badge of honor."

"But is that the whole picture?" she asked. "You have to admit that everyday life also poses a lot of stressful challenges."

"I certainly admit that we make everyday life challenging," said Dr. Alice. "As a matter of fact I had one of those challenges recently …"

✳   ✳   ✳   ✳

I was lying in my bed in a complete glacial state. Not moving. Not thinking. Not even responding when my daughter, home for the holidays, entered my bedroom and asked:

"Mom, are you okay?"

I remained frozen.

"Mom, are you sick? You look really out of it." She sat down on the bed beside me. I still did not reply.

"Mom, say something, please. I don't like it when you're quiet. It seems too strange."

So I said something. "I needed some new clothes so I went to the mall today. Alone."

It was her turn to freeze. She just sat there. Not moving. Not talking. Finally I asked: "Honey, say something please. I don't like it when you're quiet."

So she said: "I can't believe that you, a person who is like totally retail retarded went to the mall alone, two days before Christmas. Mom, I'm surprised you're still alive."

"So I am."

"But why did you go? It's not like you had an urgent need for new clothes."

"I forgot about Christmas, okay?"

"Forgot? How could you forget that?"

"I'm Jewish and it's not my holiday, is it?"

"But still Mom, Christmas stuff is everywhere."

"Let's just say I had a senior moment."

"A senior moment? Mom, you had a mummy moment."

"I did remember when I pulled into the parking lot and saw two women whacking each other with their purses over an empty parking space."

"So why didn't you just turn around and leave? You can barely deal with a mall even if it's closed."

"I know that. But then something happened." I paused hoping to add a little atmosphere to my tale.

"Mom, what happened?"

"There right before me a parking space opened up right next to the mall entrance. I took that to be a sign."

"A sign of what?"

"A miracle. Suddenly I knew how Moses felt when he saw the Red Sea parting."

"Are you trying to tell me that finding a parking space made you feel like you should go forth and conquer a Christmas crazed mall?"

"Exactly."

"But once inside, Mom, didn't you realize that you couldn't handle it or did you encounter a burning bush telling you to go forth and spend?"

"No," I said, sitting up. "But what I did see really, really puzzled me."

"What was that?"

"The merchandise. No matter where I looked I saw Santa sweaters, reindeer socks, elf slippers, mistletoe sweatshirts and underwear brimming with turtle doves. I don't get it. Don't you think there are people who really dislike what has happened to their holiday? How would I feel at Passover if stores sold matzo ball slippers or sweatshirts decorated with The Ten Plagues?"

"Mom, relax, you are never going to see that."

"But I never see people wear the other stuff either. Do you?"

"Not very often," said my daughter, looking straight at me, "and that's a really good thing or else. You would probably love wearing reindeer sox." I let that comment slide because a retarded retail shopper should never argue with a teen-age consumer authority. Instead I asked, "Haven't you ever wondered what happens to all this stuff?"

"No. Why should I?"

"Because it's a mystery, a really perplexing one. Do people give it to charities that ship it overseas? Are there whole villages in Africa or nomads in Siberia wandering around in elf slippers and reindeer socks?"

"Mom, there are no African villages or nomads in Siberia running around in elf slippers and reindeer socks!"

"Then where does all the Christmas paraphernalia go?"

"I don't know!"

"I have an idea. Maybe all the stuff gets shipped to the Middle East where they can wear it under burqas. That might explain why we never see any of it."

"Mom, who cares about this?"

"I care because 10,000 years from now some archaeologist may uncover all this paraphernalia and publish a famous paper describing us as pagans who worshipped Santa as a God of Fertility and Rudolph, with his nose so bright, as our God of the Grape. And that's not the only reason. I had a bit of a mishap with some Christmas merchandise."

"What happened?"

"Well," I said sitting up so I could add body language to the story that I was about to share. "I was standing in the mall's biggest department store, staring at a table piled high with singing Santa Claus boxers."

"What song do they sing?"

"*Santa Claus is Coming to Town*. Now, maybe it's just the way my mind works, but singing male underwear doesn't work for me. Is that really how one wants to spread the holiday spirit?"

"That is a bit disturbing," she agreed.

"I was really taken aback. I was so bothered that I didn't notice a woman behind me swinging an enormous shopping bag. I stepped back only to have her huge shopping bag accidentally knock me forward into the display of singing boxers. The next thing I knew I was lying amongst a dozen pairs of undies all crooning: *You better not cry, You better not shout ... Santa Claus is coming to town!*"

*   *   *   *

"I can't believe that you had a Christmas caroling experience with a stack of warbling underwear," she said.

"It was a one of a kind experience," said Dr. Alice.

"Yes, but I still think …"

"Yes?"

"While we may be asking for some of the stress we face every day, doesn't that story also show how nerve-racking life can be? Today, even the holiday season can be traumatic."

"Yes, but who created the trauma?" asked Dr. Alice. "I don't think we can blame Santa Claus, can we?"

"You have a point there."

"I also want to make another point. We aren't designed to handle all this constant stress. Our bodies were intended to handle stress as an occasional physical threat or a brief episode of danger, like gearing up to fight a wooly mammoth."

"At least that's one stress we don't have to face today," she said.

"But I think what we face is worse than wooly mammoths: the constant pressures that we have created. And all this pressure is taking a tremendous toll on our health. If you recall, I already mentioned that at least 70% of all disease is associated with stress?"

"I do remember," she said.

"And that may be a low estimate. A study found that 85% of health complaints at medical office visits were related to stress.[24] The good news is that there are a couple of things we can do about this. First, we can simply choose to stop inhaling all this stress. It's okay to once again be able to say:

Greeter #1: Hi, how are you?

Greeter #2: I'm fine, thanks. How are you?

Second, we need to start embracing more humor and laughter in our lives because humor not only triggers amazing health benefits, it actually acts to diminish the body's negative response to stress. And that's why I call it The Story of Stress and Disease and How Humor Gives It a Happy Ending."

"Is it one of your amusing stories?" she asked.

"Oh no," said Dr. Alice. "This story took many years and many people. But before I tell it, I first want to ask you a question: How are you?"

She smiled as she said: "I'm fine, thanks. How are you?"

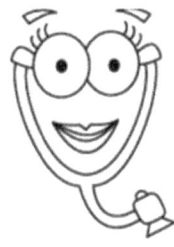

5. *The Story of Stress and Disease and How Humor Gives It a Happy Ending*

"Knowing where to start a story is never easy," said Dr. Alice. "But I think I'll begin The Story of Stress and Disease and How Humor Gives It a Happy Ending with Hans Selye."

"Hans Selye? That sounds like the guy who wrote fairy tales."

"That was Denmark's Hans Christian Anderson," said Dr. Alice. "Dr. Selye was a Canadian physician and research scientist. Although, when he first wrote in a prestigious journal that stress might be associated with disease, many called his idea a fairy tale."

"How times have changed," she said.

"They have," said Dr. Alice, "but back in 1936 when Dr. Selye first suggested this, many scoffed at the idea that stress could negatively effect your heart or your immune system."

"So this once was a truly radical idea?"

"Yes, but it became more than an idea. Dr. Selye, along with others, researched and published findings that supported this theory.[25] In time, people finally came to accept that stress can make the body more susceptible to illness."

"Did Dr. Selye live long enough to get the recognition he deserved?"

"Yes, he did," said Dr. Alice. "He lived well into the 1980's and had the satisfaction of seeing his theory become so well accepted and researched that there is now general agreement that stress can play a major role in the top three causes of death: heart disease, cancer and stroke. Together, these diseases take a huge toll on our health and on our healthcare budget. That's why scientists today continue to study the complexities of the mental and physical consequences of stress."

"So we still don't have all the answers?" she asked.

"No, we don't have all the answers," said Dr. Alice. "However, we do have enough information to know we should actively be trying to reduce anxiety levels yet most people still don't take to heart how stress can damage a body."

"I heard that double entendre," she said.

"I'm glad you heard it but if you're like most people, you won't heed it," said Dr. Alice. "I never hear anyone say, 'I've got to stop stressing. It's damaging my heart.'"

"I never hear that either," she said.

"However some people did take Dr. Selye's theory seriously to heart. One in particular made headlines doing it. His name was Norman Cousins."

"I think I've heard of him," she said. "Didn't he get some weird disease and then cure himself by laughing?"

"That's him," said Dr. Alice. "He was also the well-known editor of the widely read magazine, *The Saturday Review*, and an advocate for world peace. He was awarded the Peace Medal from the United Nations in 1971."

"He accomplished all that? What I remember is the guy who laughed his illness away."

"I think he would've liked that," said Dr. Alice, "because in 1978 he developed a crippling and sometimes fatal form of arthritis. And that's when he did something that changed his life and changed the way the world looked at humor. With his doctor's consent, he checked himself out of the hospital and into a hotel where, for several months, he enjoyed one Mirthful Laughter experience after another. I don't know how many Marx Brothers movies he watched but he slowly got better while noting things like laughter gave him up to two hours of pain free sleep." [26,27]

"Didn't he write a book about this?"

"It's called *Anatomy of an Illness*. It is still considered to be a ground breaking publication and it's why some people consider him to be a pioneer in the field of Modern Therapeutic Humor."

"Why modern?" she asked.

"There's evidence that healing with humor and laughter existed in early civilizations. The ancient Greeks built outdoor amphitheatres next to healing temples or hospitals because they noticed that patients who could enjoy comedies recovered at a faster rate."

"Sign me up for that kind of hospital."

"Wouldn't that be nice," said Dr. Alice. An HMO called: Humor Maintenance Organization."

"It appears that ancient Greece was one step ahead of us," she said.

"And not just the Greeks," said Dr. Alice. "They weren't the first to use humor in healing. Some primitive tribes had a Funny Man as well as a Medicine Man for the sick because they, too, noted that humor helped people heal. What I find particularly fascinating is that these Funny Men existed in both African and Native American tribes. Remember, there were no letters, phones or televisions. They didn't even have e-mail back then. Yet, without any communication between them, both indigenous groups came up with the idea to help cure illness through humor."

"That is interesting," she said.

"Isn't it? And of course I can't forget the Old Testament where it says: *A Merry Heart doeth more good than medicine.*"

"So people have used humor to heal for centuries," she said. "Norman Cousins just kind of rediscovered it."

"He did more than that," said Dr. Alice. "He devoted the rest of his life to studying and promoting research on the interaction between our emotions, the brain and how this effects our bodies. So, unlike primitive tribes that used intuition and observation, today we know how stress negatively effects the body's function. We also know how humor counters this effect."

"This sounds complicated," she said.

"Not my version," said Dr. Alice, "because I don't want you stressing over stress! So I'll make it simple and start by asking you to come up with a common situation that makes you feel tense or annoyed. That's easy enough, right?"

"Too easy," she said. "I can think of so many things that annoy me!"

"Can't we all? But just give me one," said Dr. Alice.

"How about being put 'on hold forever' during a phone call."

"That's perfect," said Dr. Alice. "It is incredibly annoying to have to wait … and wait … and wait. I think someone needs to program a computer voice to say: *We're sorry that your call is so unimportant to us that you will now have to listen to the same recorded message 100 times before speaking with a human.*"

"I get tense just thinking about it," she said.

"And getting annoyed is just a small part of the picture," said Dr. Alice. "As you sit there holding the phone and stewing away, your emotional state activates an area in the brain called the hypothalamus which then sends a signal to another part of the brain called the pituitary gland. When the pituitary gland receives this 'stress signal' it reacts by secreting a hormone that travels through the body to two glands that sit on top of the kidneys called the adrenals. This hormone tells these glands to quickly release stress hormones into the bloodstream. Is that clear?"

"I got the picture, but not the names," she said.

"Being able to say hypothalamus, pituitary or adrenal or 'HPA' system, which is how many refer to it, is not necessary. What's important is to know that a tense emotional state activates your brain to send a message to glands in your body telling them to release stress hormones. However, I can say this in one short sentence. Are you ready?"

"I am!"

"Stress causes your body to release stress hormones," said Dr. Alice.

"Now, that's totally clear," she said. "And, I think I have heard of these hormones. Aren't they called epi-something?"

"The three main hormones released are epinephrine, norepinephrine and cortisol. However, remembering all the names isn't necessary. What you need to understand is that stress hormones give us a sudden burst of physical energy and strength. Blood sugar rises to make sure our bodies have energy to burn while blood flow increases to the leg muscles so you can run faster. However, there is a consequence for this sudden burst of power. Blood flow to crucial organs can be restricted and the immune system can be temporarily weakened."

"Isn't that an awfully large consequence for just a short burst of energy?" she asked.

"You have to understand that our bodies first developed this as a way to respond to a brief episode of danger because most stress used to be physical in nature. Primitive man didn't worry about getting into the right college, making mortgage payments or planning a retirement pension. He was more likely to worry about the occasional showdown with a wooly mammoth where he truly needed the strength and power from the release of stress hormones. And that's why today we still call the release of these hormones *the fight or flight response*. However, stress is rarely due to physical circumstances anymore."

"I have to say that I can't remember the last time I was physically frightened," she said.

"But day in and day out we constantly worry about just getting through daily routines like fighting traffic, making deadlines at work, and orchestrating a busy family life," said Dr. Alice. "Yet every time we agonize over something like an overdue credit card bill or a dropped cell phone call, our bodies still release stress hormones into our bloodstream as if we were about to face a physical danger."

"Let me get this straight," she said. "Are you saying that our bodies react in the same way to any kind of pressure whether it's physical or mental by releasing stress hormones?"

"Yes, and that's why it's such a big problem. When we angst over things all day long, our bodies react by releasing stress hormones all day long. While prehistoric man might have released stress hormones once or twice a day, nowadays it is estimated that these hormones can be released anywhere from 30 to 50 times day. And we were not designed for all this chronic fretting because every time these hormones are released they negatively impact many parts of our body."

"So, if we stress only occasionally, this isn't a big problem?" she asked.

"No, it's not," said Dr. Alice. "Our bodies are okay with an occasional stressful occurrence. However, we were not intended to constantly gripe: 'I'm stressed out!' This constant stressing has an extremely negative effect on our heart,[15,16] blood vessels,[17] gastrointestinal tract[28] and immune system.[18,19,20] Its effect on the immune system is so profound I want to spend some time discussing this."

"This sounds rather scary," she said.

"It's less scary than facing a wooly mammoth."

"Are you sure?"

"Positive," said Dr. Alice. "In fact, I'll begin by simply stating that stress negatively effects many cells and components of the immune system including the natural killer cells. Do you remember those?"

"How could I forget? They are cells that are active against cancer and they are also the ones you want to use in a horror movie, right?"

"Right! And you just gave me idea! Maybe I should have the natural killer cells lounging on a couch watching a stressful film so their ability to fight cancer may decrease. Talk about horror. However, I don't have the time to write a script or discuss all the negative effects that stress has on the immune system. But I do want to have some fun talking about cortisol, a particularly important stress hormone and it's effect on the immune system. Maybe you've heard of it? In small amounts it's an important body regulator, but in large amounts it can help shut down the body's immune response. That's why it's used in transplant patients so they won't reject their new organ."

"I have heard of it," she said.

"But now, you get to hear and see something about it. And, to add to your pleasure and excitement about this, I have brought with me a high tech device that actually demonstrates how too much cortisol can negatively effect the immune system. Here it is!" Dr. Alice then held up a small object that looked like … a snow globe.

"Is that it?" she asked.

"Yes."

"But that looks just like a snow globe."

"It is, but it's not just any snow globe. It features an underwater scene with an octopus, some fish and a sign that says Los Angeles. And when I shake it, it snows in the sea! Global warming appears to have eluded the makers of this product!"

"But what can a snow globe tell me about stress and the immune system?"

"A lot. Now, what happens when I shake it?"

"Isn't that obvious?" she asked. "The fake snow swirls around the octopus and the fish."

"And when the snow swirls, can you still see them?" asked Dr. Alice.

"Not well."

"Cortisol acts in the same manner as the fake snow. It can actually cloud up your bloodstream so your immune cells can't see well either."

"Are you saying that when I stress, my immune cells can't see any fish or octopus in my bloodstream?"

"That's one way to look at it," said Dr. Alice smiling.

"I may never look at a snow globe in the same way again," she said. "All that fake swirling snow will make me think of cortisol and stress."

"But it doesn't have to," said Dr. Alice, "because when we laugh our brain sends out a signal that shuts down the release of stress hormones. The bloodstream clears up and now our immune cells can again function well.[20]"

"So humor and stress function in opposite ways? While stress causes the hormones to be released, humor acts to diminish them?"

"Yes, and that's why it's okay to look at a snow globe," said Dr. Alice. "I can pick it up, shake it and think of a stress hormone clouding up my immune system. However, I can set it down, watch the scene clear up and think, this is how humor transforms my body. Talk about the power of joy. This small snow globe serves to remind me that I can purposefully choose to use humor and laughter to benefit my immune system."

"Do we know this for a fact?" she asked.

"Yes we do," said Dr. Alice. "Studies have confirmed this including one that showed that a Humorized group of subjects had lower circulating levels of stress hormones when compared to a group not exposed to anything funny.[20] And that's not all. It's been shown that the brain can be 'wired' for stress." [28]

"What do you mean by that?"

"When we constantly stress day in and day out, over time your brain adapts to this by learning to quickly send out signals to release stress hormones. When this adaptation of the brain occurs, it's called 'conditioning' or 'wiring' the brain for stress. And it's obviously not a good thing, is it?"

"No."

"But you or anyone else can alter or prevent this from happening by simply choosing not to stress out all the time."

"There's so much to know and think about it, Dr. Alice."

"And I've only talked about a small part of the picture. Stress and other emotions have such a profound effect on the immune system that a whole field of science has emerged to study this phenomenon. And it has quite a name. In fact, it may take you the rest of your life to learn to pronounce it."

"Is it really that long?" she asked.

"Maybe, if you're quick, you can get it out in an hour," said Dr. Alice. It's called *psychoneuroimmunology*, but it really isn't that bad if you break it down. *Psycho* refers to emotions, *neuro* means of the brain and *immunology* is the study of our immune system. Do you want to try saying it?"

"No," she said.

"That's okay," said Dr. Alice. "It's more important to understand that it refers to the powerful connection that exists between our emotions, our mind and our immune system."

"And when was this field created?" she asked.

"In the 70's. Dr. Robert Ader a researcher at the University of Rochester is credited with being the first to recognize how the immune system is effected by our emotions.[29] However, Norman Cousins brought it into the mainstream with his book about his recovery from his arthritic condition. He then devoted his life to studying the link between our emotions and health which is why the UCLA center of psychoneuroimmunology is named for him."

"A whole field and research center devoted to the emotional impact of stress, humor and health," she said.

"Yes, isn't that something," said Dr. Alice. "However what stress does to other organs is just as important. It can take a tremendous toll on the heart, blood vessels, and the GI tract."

"I do remember that stress narrows the arteries," she said.

"Up to 35%," said Dr. Alice. "This narrowing of the arteries can lead to heart disease, high blood pressure and stroke, all leading causes of death in this country."

"Now, that is scarier than a charging wooly mammoth," she said.

"It might be," said Dr. Alice, "and I still haven't even mentioned that stress may cause your GI tract to bloat and spasm leading to nausea and vomiting. It may also spur the release of inflammatory cells in the intestines, which may play a role in irritable bowel syndrome (IBS), a chronic condition that causes abdominal pain and problems in up to 15% of the population." [28]

"I've seen drug ads on television for that," she said.

"Reducing stress in people with IBS may be just as important and effective as taking drugs," said Dr. Alice. "And finally, I want to mention once again that stress plays a role in most of our major diseases. And while the epidemic of obesity is deservedly getting a lot of attention, I also think it's time to consider that the epidemic of stress needs to be considered as well."

"It sounds like the phrase 'worried to death' has never been more relevant," she said.

"We are worrying ourselves into poorer health," said Dr. Alice. "And while humor and laughter have not directly been shown to combat stroke, cancer or IBS, the fact that humor does diminish the release of stress hormones suggests that it may play an important role in combating these diseases and making us healthier. That's why I call this 'The Story of Stress and Disease and How Humor Gives It a Happy Ending.'"

"Yes, but I'm not ready for the end yet," she said. "I want to know how much humor one needs to experience."

"A study showed that just watching a funny video of their choice for 20-30 minutes daily diminished the release of stress hormones in study subjects," [20] said Dr. Alice. "And the good news is that you don't even have to laugh out loud for this happen. The same good levels of stress hormones can be found in people who simply smiled or just anticipated a joyful or funny experience as those who laughed out loud.[7] You don't have to be one of those who shriek and cackle in order to enjoy the many benefits of humor and laughter."

"Only 20-30 minutes a day?" she asked. "Isn't that the same amount of time the heart patients spent watching funny shows?"

"It's also the same amount of time needed to boost many of your immune cells," said Dr. Alice.

"20-30 minutes sounds like the magic number," she said.

"But is it magical enough to make you start wanting to treat yourself to a small, daily dose of humor? I remember that you were skeptical about adding The Feel Good Lifestyle to your own life."

"I think it is," she said. "But it will be a bit of an adjustment. It's a whole new way to take in giggling and stressing."

"Which is why I call it The Humor Revolution," said Dr. Alice.

"Whatever you call it," she said, "I think that you shouldn't just be talking with me. Honestly, you should be doing more with this. Wouldn't chit chatting with Oprah be a better way to start a Humor Revolution?"

"It's funny that you should say that," said Dr. Alice.

"Have you tried to get on Oprah?" she asked.

"Oh no. Your question just reminded me of a story I once wrote about some dreams I had of becoming famous."

"And was Oprah in the story?"

"Yes," said Dr. Alice.

"And is this a funny story you can share? I could use a break."

"It's certainly not going to release any stress hormones," said Dr. Alice …

*   *   *   *

"Boogs, what are you up to?" I practically jumped ten feet at the sound of his voice. I had been so consumed by a thought I had failed to hear my husband and daughter enter my home office.

"Just thinking," I said.

"I hope it's about dinner," said my husband.

"Dinner? I hardly ever think about that."

He sighed in agreement. "So, what are you thinking about?"

"Dad, you don't want to ask Mom that ever," said my daughter.

"Why not?"

"Because Mom has that look on her face. The one she gets when she is thinking up some insane idea."

"Her ideas are sometimes a little odd, but …"

"A little odd? Dad, maybe it's time for you to wake up and smell your wife."

"And I think," he said, "that it's time for you to go and get the take-out menus." Our daughter stomped off. I never knew pink flip-flops could make so much noise.

"She's right," I said, watching her leave. "I am having one of my insane ideas."

"Really, what is it?"

"I don't know if I am ready to share."

"Come on, tell me."

"I have decided that I don't want death to kill all thoughts of me."

"You don't want death to … Boogs, what are you saying?"

"I'm simply saying that I don't wish to spend my afterlife with the eternally forgotten."

My husband grew quiet. Very quiet. It seemed like hours passed before he asked: "Are you trying to tell me that you want to become one of the rich and famous?" I nodded. "But Boogs, how are you going to do that? I have never seen a public health doctor on the cover of 'People' magazine."

"No, but I could do something else. My Mom always used to tell me that I was the best at everything: the best student, the best dancer, even the best chewer."

"Chewer?"

"Yes, chewer. I can clearly recall her saying, 'Alice, you could be the Queen of Mastication.'"

"Boogs, having known your mom I believe you, but there's not any fame or money in mastication."

"I know. That's why I have been thinking about a famous quote by Ben Franklin: *If you would not be forgotten as soon as you are dead, either do things worth writing or write things worth reading.*"

"That's an interesting way to look at it. Are you going to do or write?"

"Do," I said, "it's so much more glamorous than writing, don't you think?"

"But what exactly will you do?"

"I don't know yet. I thought I would start by making a list of possibilities."

"You go to it, Boogs," he said, reaching down to kiss me. "And don't forget to have fun while you dream."

Have fun? Fantasize? Dream the impossible? "Well, why not was my thought as I began to make my list:

1. Become a Famous Athlete

Imagine: me as the next Tiger Woods driving a golf ball with the same skill and daring that I use to drive my Toyota Camry. Imagine: me as the next Serena Williams backhanding a tennis racket with the same skill more than strawberries at Wimbledon. Then again, imagine: me barely passing PE. Oh well, maybe I shouldn't feel bad because athletic feats, while entertaining, don't really make a difference in most people's lives. However, no one could guess that by the size of the salaries handed to sports stars. Just think of how many starving children Mother Theresa could have fed if she had been able to hit fifty home runs a year.

Time to move on.

2. Have Sex with the President of U.S.

This was a much simpler solution ... but could I do it? Probably not. My political chastity comes from my own old-fashioned belief in 'till death do us part.' The only man for me is my husband, and I work hard to keep our romance alive.

Just recently I bought an inflatable, singing boat called *Titanic II* designed for use in the bedroom. Every weekend I blow it up, stand on the bow with my eyes closed and arms flying with my hubby right behind me. Entwined together we listen to the boat sing, "My Heart Will Go On." After experiencing that kind of passion with my spouse, how could I ever think of anyone else?

Time to move on.

3. Become a Body Builder then Actor then Governor

Who wouldn't like the idea of following in Arnold Schwarzenegger's footsteps? Pumping iron wearing a thong bikini can't be all that hard, and Hollywood loves a well-muscled woman. And after becoming a famous actress, the transition to politics will be a cinch. Why? It's because an actor's job is very similar to a politician's. They both read from scripts. The only real difference is that the scripts an actor reads are called screenplays, while the scripts a politician reads are eventually called history.

But, realistically, could I do it all? While I had no qualms about my acting genius, I did question my ability to create masses of muscles by lifting my one and a half pound binoculars while birding. And would I, with my penchant for art house movies, be able to attract voters? I had grave doubts because I believe that the type of movies Arnold made were absolutely key to his election. Such titles as *Conan the Barbarian, True Lies* and *The Terminator* gave him tremendous credibility when he decided to turn politician.

Perhaps I needed to downsize my ambitions. Forget the body building and politicking and concentrate on the more realistic goal.

4. Become a Movie Star

Bingo. Finally, an attainable goal. Just stand in front of a camera and pretend to be someone else. With a bit of luck, I might even become the next Marilyn Monroe and have my name enshrined in a sidewalk star on Hollywood Boulevard where thousands of people from all over the world will walk all over me. Dreams aside, I truly believed that I could make it. In me, directors would find a fresh look, a fresh face and of course, fresh talent. How could I be sure? Just look around. There are no flabby, wrinkly gray-haired women on either the big or little screen. Hollywood must be desperate for people like me.

I was so excited by the idea of being "discovered" that after dinner that night I shared my optimism with my kids.

"You think you can become a what?" asked my daughter.

"An actress," I said casually.

"An actress? Sure, Mom," said my son.

"Mom has probably just joined some amateur acting group that performs skits at nursing homes or something. Isn't that right?" asked my daughter.

"No, that's not right. I am considering a career move to the big or little screen."

Neither of them said a word for a long, long time. Finally my daughter said: "Mom, maybe you need to do some re-thinking or maybe just thinking. The only possible thing you could do is host a cooking show."

"If they call it *Torch*," said my son.

"What a perfect title," said my daughter. "Mom could demonstrate her technique for blackening anything. Just place it in a pot, turn on the stove and forget about it until it mutates or explodes."

"She could even feature a live band on her show and hire me," said my son, an aspiring musician. "Every time she takes out a fresh ingredient we could play the *Funeral March*."

While my culinary skills have involved feats such as scorching the kitchen ceiling, I absolutely refused to be relegated to the Food Network. I wanted to star in my own sitcom. I let my two genetic aberrations know this.

My son laughed. My daughter didn't.

"Mom," she said, "The only sitcom you could ever star in would be 'No Sex and the City.'"

"What?" I shrieked.

"Mom, look at you. Your face is like, old, and your arms jiggle when you move."

"So does her butt," added my son.

"But Hollywood needs women with wrinkles and jiggles!"

"Mom, what could possibly give you that idea?" asked my daughter.

"Isn't it obvious? You never see women like me on TV. Television must be desperate for genuine, middle-aged flesh. I am destined to hit it big because I will be new. Exciting. Different."

"I won't argue the different," said my son, rising and leaving the room.

"Where's he going?" I asked.

"Back to reality," said my daughter. "You should follow him. So, listen up Mom."

"I'm listening."

"Do you have any idea why the big studios are patrolled by armed security guards?"

"No."

"Hollywood executives are determined to keep women like you off the screen."

"Why?"

"They feel it's their job to protect the public from the fact that people age."

"They do?"

"So, Mom, unless you are willing to have plastic surgery and Botox, stay away from film or television studios. I have heard that security guards are under strict orders to shoot tranquilizer darts at anyone trying to enter who looks over forty."

Oh well, I guess I was just never going to have the chance to become the next Julia Roberts. I was sad, but not crushed. In my heart I knew that author, Dr. Lawrence Peter, was right when he suggested that most screen celebrities are: *Hero today, gone tomorrow.*

With no desire to be treated like an escaped wild animal, I decided that it was time to forget doing something glamorous. Instead, I would try to write my way into a literary hall of fame. Frankly, the more I thought about it, the more I felt this was the right choice. Isn't fame easier said than done? So I crossed out my first list and began work on my second:

1. The Political Book

Now that's a hot item. People just can't get enough books on how America is messing up America. But could I write one? Did I have the political savvy, insight and skill of Bob Woodward or Monica Lewinsky? Probably not.

Moving Ahead.

2. A Novel Novel

Who hasn't dreamed of writing the great American novel and seeing one's name on a bestseller list? But could I do this? The best way to find out was a short test run. I decided to try the sexually tempestuous love story first. With romance novelist Danielle Steele in mind I wrote: *She realized that his pulsating phallic manhood was about to take off like a rocket so she asked, "Have you recently been tested for HIV? And if you haven't, could you please wear five condoms?"*

Somehow I don't think that's how Ms. Steele made her fortune. I guess being a public health doctor is a real liability when it comes to bodice ripping romance.

I could still try writing in another genre. How about a thriller with religious and symbolic references? Could I emulate Dan Brown, author of *The Da Vinci Code*? I could try: *Only a very few knew that Picasso drew faces with missing parts as a sign that a secret underground circumcision society called 'The Clip-inati' was trying to take over the Catholic Church.*

That sounded too much like a current popular book. Maybe I just don't have the thriller instinct.

Fresh out of ideas I decided I needed to check out other literary possibilities at a bookstore. But not just any bookstore. I planned on trying out a new "super-sized" one that had recently opened. I was already curious about it because it had such an interesting name: *Barnyards and Noodles*.

I had no trouble finding the store since it covered ten city blocks. They weren't kidding around when they called it "supersized." Then again, they needed the space for the coffee lounge, sushi bar, smoothie stand, desserterie, salad bar, candy corner and, of course, *Barnyards and Noodles'* two signature attractions: a petting zoo and a noodle kitchen. I was just wondering how to manage the mile long store when I saw a tram called *Desire*. How cute. My search would have to wait. I hopped on the tram heading towards the *Barnyard*. I could never resist a chance to pet baby animals.

The short ride took me to a small corral that contained a few small chicks, pig-lets and two adorable baby goats that won me over. I had a great time cooing, stroking and feeding them special goat wafers. It took the appearance of a pun-gent puddle to finally motivate me to leave. Waving good-bye to the two cuties, I closed the gate and asked the keeper one last question: "Do they have names?"

"Oh, yes," she replied. "We call them War and Peace." She then smiled and handed me a complimentary bookmark that said: *Barnyards and Noodles, The Place To Go For Petting and Reading*.

After washing my hands I hopped back on a tram headed towards the Culi-nary Court. All those goat wafers had revved up my appetite. I treated myself to a salad followed by my usual decaf single shot low-fat vanilla latte. With drink in hand, I finally set off to check out the books. I began by noting the unusual, yet helpful displays. Forget about a fiction section simply arranged by author. Here, novels were divided into much more logical headings like *Happy Endings, Surprise Endings,* and *Books Where You Will Never Get the Ending*. The non-fiction section was even more unique, featuring a self-help section five blocks long. I couldn't help asking a worker:

"Why do you need such a huge collection?"

He looked at me like I was nuts. "This is LA, Lady."

I could have drifted around for hours, but I did have a mission to accomplish. I started my official search for literary fame near the sushi bar. It turned out to be an excellent choice because only a few yards away I noticed a sign that said: *Oprah Books*. I knew that I had hit gold. Many people already know that Oprah Winfrey, arguably the most famous talk show host in the country, recommends a book every month. Not only does she inspire people to read, but every last one of her choices became a bestseller. Talk about instant celebrity status. All I had to do was write a book that Oprah couldn't resist. With determination, daring and latte in hand, I walked right up to that table and one by one waded through dozens of books she had gilded. It didn't take long to realize that one kind of book hooked her every time. She loved to read "victim books." While it may seem hard to believe, almost every single book I looked at focused on overcoming hardships like kidnapping, alcoholism, mental illness, marital infidelity, abuse, abandonment, the holocaust, slavery, etc.

Whatever her reasons for liking walking disasters, I left that store one happy camper. All I had to do was go home and write the greatest victim book of the 21st century. While some might be daunted by this task, I modestly admit that I came up with a synopsis that would have Oprah drooling. My book would tell the tale of a kidnapping victim left in a Wal-Mart who was subsequently rescued by a mental patient with no arms. She then sets out on a journey to Africa to find her roots and the hippopotamus that will change her life. On the way she falls in love with a pilot who marries her but then cruelly abandons her for a movie star turned missionary who is searching all of Africa for a mosquito that will cure AIDS. Devastated, our heroine becomes an alcoholic who eventually gives birth to Siamese triplets. Despite all of this, she eventually becomes President of the United States and does away with the Electoral College.

Could a story be more thrilling? I even loved my title: *The Pilot's Wife's Hippo*. How could I not end up on Oprah? And I couldn't keep all this excitement to myself, so I shared my budding story with my family. At least my husband kept his comments to the plausibility of the plot.

"Boogs," he asked, "it's not clear who gets her pregnant. Is it the husband who abandons her or the hippopotamus?"

However, my daughter's comment went beyond the story line. "Mom, there is only one way Oprah would have you as a guest on her show."

"What way is that?" I asked.

"You would have to be dubbed." My son agreed.

Sadly, I realized that it was time to give up my fantasy of aspiring fame and glory. Yet, before closing the door on my dream I did one last thing. I looked up the formal definition of the word celebrity and much to my surprise I read: "someone held up for acclaim." How strange. This phrase did not conjure up images of movie stars, athletes or famous authors. It made me think of the remarkable people that are important in my life, my family and friends. These are the ones that I hold up for "acclaim" since I bask in their good deeds, their kindness and their generosity. How nice it was to come to the conclusion that I will, after all, be pleased to coexist with the eternally forgotten.

✳ ✳ ✳ ✳

"So you never did write The Pilot's Wife Hippo?" she asked.

"No, but I sure had fun thinking about it which means that my heart got a boost, my immune system revved up and I was left feeling optimistic and relaxed."

"There are so many reasons to be smile and laugh more," she said.

"Yes, but it's okay not to remember all the details. What's important is that you understand why it's so important to smile and laugh."

"You've made that clear."

"So does that mean you are ready to start being Humorized?" asked Dr. Alice.

"Aren't we already doing that?"

"I've begun by encouraging you to activate your Humor Antennae and tune in Humorvision and making sure you understand all the amazing mind and body benefits of humor. Now it's time to look at how humor can make your daily life more enjoyable and emotionally satisfying."

"Laugh more, stress less?"

"Exactly," said Dr. Alice, "and what better place to start than by showing you how humor can relieve stress from everyday annoyances to complex emotional issues."

"Is that possible?" she asked.

"Yes, in fact, human beings have been using humor as a coping mechanism since prehistoric times. There is even written documentation that stressed out cave men used Jewish humor when faced with a charging, wooly mammoth."

"And am I supposed to believe that?"

"No," said Dr. Alice, "but I do hope you'll believe what else I have to say about humor as a stress reliever."

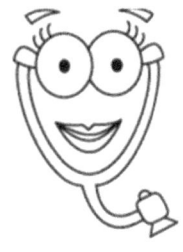

6. Coping Humor I
The Red-Caped Stress Reliever

"We've just looked at how humor can lower the level of stress hormones and make us healthier," said Dr. Alice. "Now it's time to look at how Coping Humor can help us handle emotional stress and make us happier."

"Coping Humor?"

"When you actively choose to use Mirthful Humor or Laughter to ease or deflect stress, you're using Coping Humor" said Dr. Alice. "And while humor may not be able to change the stress or a challenging situation, it can give you a lovely, momentary break. And just having that small break can do wonders. You can return to the problem with a new perspective and fresh energy. It's a powerful tool that can be used in many circumstances. For example, remember how you said that 'being out on hold forever stressed you out?'"

"It always does," she said.

"Coping Humor works great for Man-made Stress. However it can also ease the anxiety of more complex and emotional challenges."

"So it's a way to relieve stress from daily problems to more complex issues?"

"That's exactly what it is," said Dr. Alice. "What it's not is a treatment for chronic anxiety. While humor and laughter may be a wonderful addition for people with ongoing mental problems, it's not an accepted mode of management. You can use Coping Humor to help ease the stress on 'being put on hold' but if you end up being 'put on hold' for a week, and subsequently have a nervous breakdown, you need more than humor!"

"I would think so," she said.

"But the good news is that most of our stress does come from daily problems that respond well to Coping Humor," said Dr. Alice. "I even used it to survive shopping at a furniture store the size of Florida ..."

＊　　＊　　＊　　＊

"Mom," said my daughter. "When are we going shopping for that new bedroom set that you have been promising me forever?"

I got the hint. "This week?"

"Okay, tomorrow," she said, before mentioning a store where she wanted to go. I didn't catch the name, it was so unusual, so I asked her to repeat it.

"That's a hard word to pronounce," I said after hearing it again. "What a mouthful of vowels. Is it Japanese?"

"Actually, it's a Swedish company," said my daughter.

"Why would a Swedish store have a Japanese name?"

"Mom, it isn't Japanese."

"It sure doesn't sound Swedish."

"How would you know?"

"I know some Swedish words, like sockerkaka, pepperkaka, and jordgubbstarta."

"What do they mean, Mom?"

"Sugar cake, gingersnaps and strawberry torte."

"Mom, you may know dessert names in every language but no one is going to call a furniture store 'Sugar Cake.'"

"Why not? Sockerkaka sounds a lot better than what it's called."

I never did get the name of that store down, but that didn't matter. What mattered was that my daughter had assured me that it was inexpensive. Imagine my surprise when my son appeared astonished at our destination.

"Mom, are you really going there?" he asked, while I was standing by the front door waiting for his sister to change from school clothes into a shopping outfit.

"Why shouldn't I go there?" I asked. "I hear it's a popular place to buy furniture."

"Popular is right. The guy who owns it is richer than Bill Gates, but I don't think it's for you."

I was touched by his concern, but I wasn't worried. I can get anxious in a large supermarket or a big mall, but I have never had a problem buying furniture. If you need a couch, you walk into a showroom, pick one out, buy it and arrange for delivery. No big deal.

However, I never got a chance to reassure him. At that moment his sister joined us asking: "Are you ready to go?"

Before I could answer, my son pounced. "Are you really taking Mom to that store?"

"I can't drive," said his sister, "and anyway, Mom will be fine. I'll be with her the whole time."

"Fine? I ought to call Channel Four News. This could make quite a story."

I didn't know what to make of that conversation, but it didn't stop us from leaving and traveling a lot further than I bargained for. We were still searching for our destination when I spied a massive, purplish blue building with no windows.

"Can you believe the size of that building?" I said. "It must be several blocks long. I wonder what's in it."

"I know what's in it, Mom. Furniture."

"Really? Is it some kind of warehouse?"

"No."

I hit the brake, pulled the car over and turned to my daughter. I suddenly understood what my son was talking about. "Is that it?"

"Yes."

"I can't go in there. That's the scariest building I ever saw."

"Mom, thousands of people go in there every day."

"Thousands may go in, but how many come out? I bet half the people pictured on milk cartons were last seen here."

"Mom, it's just a big store, okay?"

"Big? It's more than big. They should call it 'The Blue Hole.' What do they need all that space for anyway?"

"They sell all kinds of things."

"Like what? Jumbo jets? Pre-fab office buildings? The state of Florida?"

"Mom, just calm down and park the car because we're going in."

The Furniture Goddess had spoken. I followed the long, winding loop into the parking lot that appeared to go forever. Unfortunately, I found a space and parked. I was then dragged from the car.

"You should've warned me," I said, as I followed my daughter towards the one entrance and exit.

"You wouldn't have come if I had told you," she said, as we passed through the door and onto the escalator.

"You would've still talked me into it but at least I would've brought some pro-visions, like water, snacks and a sleeping bag. We could be here for days."

"Mom, just stay close to me and I'll have us out in no time."

It's hard to stay close to someone who steps off an escalator shrieking, "That's so hot!" and then disappears into the deep, dark caverns of furniture hell. Who did she see? Johnny Depp? Will Smith? No. She saw something better: a shock-ing pink sofa.

"Honey," I said, catching up to her, "I thought we were going to stay together."

"Mom, I can't be thinking about staying together when I see the couch of my dreams."

"But we aren't buying a couch."

"Mom, look at it. It's so hot."

I looked and tried to feel the heat but nothing happened; not even one little fiery flash. Maybe that was a good thing. Somebody had to stay cool and ask: "But where will you put it? You only have room for a bed, a dresser and a desk."

"I can buy a lofted bed. It's like a bunk bed without the bottom bunk so I can put the desk underneath it. Problem solved."

"I guess that solves the space problem, but is a lofted bed comfortable?"

"Mom, I can't believe that you are talking about being comfortable, like, who cares? My room will look so cool with a lofted bed and a hot pink couch."

I couldn't say no to all that excitement. "Okay, okay," I said. She squealed and hugged me while I turned practical.

"How do we buy it?" My daughter didn't know so off we went in search of someone to ask.

One hour later we finally found a young lady standing by a computer wearing the same purple-blue color as the outside of the building. I approached her with a smile but I did not get one in return. Frankly, I have seen mannequins display more animation. However she did answer our question.

"There's a slip of paper by every item saying if it's in stock. If it is, write down the number and take it with you to the warehouse. All the items are arranged by number."

"I don't think you understood me," I said. "I don't want to pick up my own furniture. I want to have it delivered."

"You can't do that here. Everyone has to pick up their items at the warehouse, take them to the cash register and pay. If you want them delivered, you then take the items over to a different counter to arrange for delivery."

"You mean we have to haul all our own furniture out of the warehouse? How can we do that?"

"We supply you with large shopping carts."

"Shopping carts? We're talking couches and beds!"

"The furniture comes boxed up in small pieces. You put it together at home."

"Are you saying that we have to assemble the items ourselves?"

"Yes."

"How long does it take to assemble?"

"That depends on what you are buying."

"How about a bed frame or a dresser?"

"A bed may come in only six or eight pieces, but a dresser, that could take a while because it comes in many pieces. It took my friend three days to put one together."

"Three days?"

"Mom," said my daughter, "I'm sure Dad and I can do this in no time at all."

"Does Dad know about this?" I asked.

"No, but he likes building things. He'll be cool about it."

I wasn't so sure my husband would enjoy spending his entire weekend assembling furniture, but all I could say was: "I still don't see how a couch can come in a box."

"The couch comes assembled. You will have to tip it on its side to fit it into the shopping cart," said the woman.

I was stunned. How could a furniture store that makes you cart around your own couch make someone richer than Bill Gates? Obviously, there must be people who help you.

"No," was the answer. "There is no one to help."

"No oxen? No yaks? Not even one little sherpa?" I asked.

"I know we don't sell oxygen or yachts, but we may have shampoo. Do you want me to check?"

"No, that's okay. I'm just babbling. It's a bit overwhelming to think of furniture as Legos for adults."

"I have never thought of it before," said the sales girl, "but you're right except Legos come in much prettier boxes. Ours are just brown."

"How surprising," I answered. "I expected the boxes to be the same purplish-blue as your shirt and the store. Someone missed a marketing extravaganza there, unless of course, colored boxes are in the works?"

"I don't think so," said the girl.

"That's too bad. Is it because they are too busy coming up with a theme park to go along with the store?"

"A theme park?"

"Absolutely," I said. "Legos built Legoland. Why don't you build Furnitureland? It could be great. Just think of the rides you could have: The Haunted Warehouse, Mr. Chair's Wild Ride, and your own version of my favorite ride at Disneyland. Imagine sailing in a boat through all the showrooms gazing in awe at the mechanical sales people in their purplish-blue outfits who are kicking up their legs and singing: *It's a small store after all, it's a small store after all, it's a small store after all, it's a small, small store ...*"

"Mom! Stop singing!" I ceased my crooning and let my daughter drag me away. "You really need to get a grip ... Oh, that's so cool!"

So much for me needing to get a grip. My daughter was practically swooning at a desk that dared the color pink to be all it can be.

"Mom, I can see it all now: a pink couch, a pink desk with a black desk chair, a black dresser and a black lofted bed frame. To tie it all together I will add a pink comforter and black sheets. My room will look so cool and so hot."

What could I say? The truth? That her room will look like a brothel? Oh well, I guess it really didn't matter. I smiled and followed her as she went from room to room to room to room to room to room writing down the code numbers of the furniture she desired. I just tried to keep from hyperventilating as we collected tag after tag after tag until we were finally ready to head downstairs to the warehouse. But instead of moving, I froze. By now, more than two hours had passed since we had parked the car. I was tired, hungry and pinkified

"Mom," my daughter asked, "are you okay?"

"No," I said. "I am not okay. I am totally freaked out at the thought of going downstairs to haul hot pink furniture around on a barge with wheels. I need a break."

"I hear there's a cafeteria somewhere in here. Maybe we could go chill there awhile. I wouldn't mind trying the Swedish meatballs."

It took only twenty minutes to find it. Surprisingly, it was smallish and not crowded so we simply walked up to the counter to check out the choices. While I was saddened by the dearth of sockerkaka, they did at least sell Swedish meatballs. And as I gazed at those small, circular balls, I suddenly knew what would help me survive this ordeal.

I waved my hand at a server to get her attention and asked: "Is this food for display only?" She looked puzzled so I clarified the question. "What I want to know is, can I buy the meatballs I see in front of me? Or do I need to write down a number for them, go down to a corral, find a cow, kill it, load it onto a shopping cart the size of a barge, then haul it over to the check-out counter where I will pay for it, butcher it and then cook it myself?"

*   *   *   *

"I can't believe you said that," she said.

"But I'm so glad I did," said Dr. Alice. "Because that brief moment of humor temporarily lifted me out of a situation that was beginning to overwhelm me."

"I like the visual of 'lifting you out.'"

"I like it, too," said Dr. Alice, "which is why I like to see humor and laughter as a big hook that can suddenly descend and lift you up, up and away from the stress of a situation. Of course, this Humor Hook has to eventually put you back down, but by that time you have hopefully had a chance to breathe deeply, refresh your outlook, and if you are fortunate, return with a new perspective or insight on the problem. In my case, the Humor Hook gave me a laugh that lowered my stress level and infused me with enough energy and courage that I was able to face the ordeal waiting for me at the checkout stand."

"While I do like the image of the Humor Hook lifting you up, Dr. Alice, all this talk also brings to mind another visual that you could use that's a bit more exciting."

"Exciting?"

"Yes," she said. "You like to use Coping Humor to rescue you from stressful situations?"

"I do."

"Then, instead of a hook, why not think of Coping Humor as some hunky, red-caped crusader that dives down to temporarily sweep you up in his massive arms. Isn't that more appealing?"

"It might be," said Dr. Alice, laughing. "And it is a great visual: Coping Humor as a superhero."

"So you like it?" she asked.

"How could I not love the idea of some hunky guy wearing tight tights and a red cape sporting smiley faces rescuing me from stress? I'm not dead, am I?"

"And you have to admit," she added, "it's a perfect image for a revolution, isn't it?"

"I don't know about that. As much as I love to think of Coping Humor with bulging thighs and massive shoulders, I don't know if The Red-Caped Stress

Reliever fits into my Humor Revolution. If I use him, people might have a hard time taking Coping Humor seriously."

"So I have to kiss him good-by?"

"Oh no," said Dr. Alice. "You can use his superpowers any time you want. However, when I give a talk, I think I'll play it safe and stick with The Humor Hook. However from now on I'll at least think of The Humor Hook wearing a small red cape."

"With smiley faces?"

"Why not? That might help reinforce the message that The Humor Hook can be as powerful as a hunky guy in tight tights."

"While I like the idea of Coping Humor, Dr. Alice, I still have a feeling that using it might be more difficult than it seems. We're having a lot of fun talking about it, but I'm still not sure that I could easily use it. Look at how you diffused your stressful experience at the Swedish store with the Japanese name. I don't think just anyone, including me, could spontaneously come up with the way you made fun of the situation at the cafeteria."

"I'm so glad you brought this up because you are not the only person to question their ability to find the lighter side of a situation. However, I wouldn't worry too much. The one thing that always amazes me is how funny and clever most people are when given the chance. And I know that you are not the exception."

"I'm not?"

"Who brought up the red-caped superhero?" asked Dr. Alice.

"I did."

"So don't be afraid to tap into your inner humor. It's always waiting to play with you."

"A play date with humor?" she asked.

"That's a great way to look at it, especially if it helps you realize that my use of humor at the Swedish store with the Japanese name was not totally spontaneous."

"It wasn't?"

"No," said Dr. Alice. "I had my first hint of something stressful when my son appeared to be so astonished at my destination. Then I saw the size of the building and that was certainly more than a hint. Even before I entered the door to furniture hell, my Humor Antennae had already alerted my Humor Hook that it might be needed to help me survive the ordeal. I also knew that I needed to reach for the Humor Hook before I was totally overwhelmed by the stress of the situation. It couldn't help me if I was passed out on that hot pink sofa, could it?"

"No, but if you had a tag on someone might have bought you," she said.

"No, no. First they would have to write my number down, buy the box of me and then assemble me at home."

"Of course," she said, "what was I thinking?"

"So I was already thinking through my options as I entered the store and making fun of the situation seemed perfect especially since Coping Humor doesn't have to be sophisticated. It just needs to amuse you."

"And you did have plenty of time to look around to see what could amuse you."

"Yes, but more importantly, I knew I was heading into a stressful situation and instead of just being bombarded by it, I chose to support myself with humor. In fact, we are often faced with situations that are stressful and unavoidable and we can sometimes plan ahead of time to use Coping Humor to help us through them. It's what I usually do when going to see a doctor."

She cracked up. "That's a pretty funny thing for you to pick, Dr. Alice."

"But it's a perfect circumstance to use Coping Humor since you know ahead of time that you may need to use it. Not only does one worry about what might be found, we are often asked to wait forever. I used to get really bothered every time I saw my knee doctor because the wait is always so long and I can't do anything to change this. I've even tried calling ahead to see if he's running late, but the office always says that he's on schedule even when he's two hours behind. Of course I take a book with me, but the book can't diffuse the aggravation. Finally, I decided that instead of just sitting in that freezing cold, sterile examining room feeling my blood pressure rise to alarming levels, I would find some humor to help me cope."

"And did you?" she asked.

"Yes. It was surprisingly easy. I just looked around the room and suddenly I found myself asking, isn't it ironic that when you most need a nurturing environment, all you get is a cold, barren room perfumed with antiseptic smells? Who came up with the idea that hospitals and clinics should be like this?"

"And did you find out?"

"No, but I came up with my own idea of how it must have happened. I think two powerful people once had a conversation that went like this:

* * * *

Power Person #1: Guess what, old man? We've been selected to design buildings for the sick!

Power Person #2: Really? That could be tricky, couldn't it?

PP#1: Tricky? Why do you think that?

PP#2: Because the sick are often scared, anxious, and overwhelmed.

PP#1: But that makes it easy, you old fool. All we have to do is design something to reflect those feelings. So we need to make the buildings cold and forbidding.

PP#2: Do you really think so? Actually, I was thinking of something warm and welcoming like a big cottage. Maybe with a bakery attached so people can bask in the scent of freshly baked chocolate brownies. Wouldn't that be comforting?

PP#1: No, no, you are totally off base. I insist the buildings look like the inside of a fridge.

PP#2: A fridge?

PP#1: Yes, you idiot. A fridge keeps food in top shape. Why not people?

*   *   *   *

"And now every time I go see any doctor," said Dr. Alice, "I just imagine myself as a nice piece of cheese or a carton of yogurt and that makes the long wait a lot easier."

"And do you prefer to think of yourself as a hard cheese like cheddar or something soft, like Brie?"

"Definitely something soft," said Dr. Alice. "However, all joking aside, are you beginning to see that if you just allow your imagination free rein and rev up your sense of fun, you will find Coping Humor easy to use?"

"I still think it may take me awhile to develop my confidence, let alone my humor skills."

"And there's nothing wrong with that," said Dr. Alice. "It's not like you have a timeline or a test to pass and besides, we're not talking rocket comics here. All you have to do is start looking around you to find one teeny tiny bit of silliness or amusement. You'll be surprised at how quickly this becomes part of your life. In fact, why don't we try it now?"

"Now?"

"Why not? You give me an example of something that recently happened to you where you needed a Humor Hook. It doesn't have to be anything complicated. Just pick something simple."

She thought for a moment and then said: "Okay. I went to a wedding recently that turned out to be quite stressful."

"That's not surprising. Weddings today can be stressful for the guests and especially for the bride. Frankly, I wouldn't be surprised if honeymoon suites soon offer heart shaped bathtubs filled with Prozac."

"Well, I don't know if the bride was stressed, but I was," she said. They crammed 250 people into a reception room meant to hold 200. It was so uncomfortable. My husband and I could barely move."

"So the scene looked more like a people compressor than a party?"

"You're right," she said smiling. "It did."

"And did that give you sardine envy?"

"Sardine envy?"

"When I am bunched together in a small space with other people I always have sardine envy," said Dr. Alice. "At least when they're all packed together, they're dead."

She laughed. "I don't know about that. I have never really thought about being a seafood corpse."

"Then maybe the event could make you think about the dinner being a no carbs meal," said Dr. Alice, "since nobody could afford to put on an ounce in that space."

"That thought didn't cross my mind, but it should have," she said shaking her head.

"Did you consider crawling under the tables to reach your designated one?"

"That might have worked, but we didn't try it."

"You can consider crawling around at your next crammed event," said Dr. Alice. "Or maybe by then, you will feel so comfortable using Coping Humor you'll have come up with some ideas and tricks of your own."

"Tricks?"

"Yes, tricks," said Dr. Alice. "Over the years I have developed a few little humor games or tricks that I can use over and over again to help me alleviate stress."

"And do you pull these tricks out of a black hat?"

"No, I get them from that hunky, red-caped stress relieving superhero."

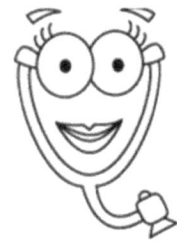

Laughing with Dr. Alice
Experience the Power of Joy

7. Coping Humor II
Can Laughter Make Parting a Sweeter Sorrow?

"Over the years I have developed a few tricks or perhaps I should call them 'strategies' that I use over and over again when faced with certain stressful circumstances," said Dr. Alice. "I have a favorite that anyone can easily use. I call it the *just pretend to be stuck in a Woody Allen movie trick.*"

"And how does it work?" she asked.

"Why don't I give you an example. It's a particularly relevant one because, it too, occurred at a wedding."

"Was the wedding also overcrowded?"

"No, the space was fine."

"Then what was the problem?"

"I'm not sure there is a word to describe what I experienced, but at least I was carrying my favorite Coping Humor trick in my beach bag."

"You carried a beach bag?" she asked. "To a wedding?"

"Believe me, carrying a beach bag was the most normal thing that happened at this wedding …"

*   *   *   *

"I am completely confused," I said to my daughter while staring at a wedding invitation.

My daughter grabbed the invitation from me and read: *Black Tie Beach Wear*. "How cool," she said, "a wedding with a *Surf 'n' Silk* theme."

"The bride and groom are avid surfers but *Black Tie Beach Wear*? I still haven't figured out if *Dressy Casual* means dressy or casual."

"Mom, it's like, so obvious."

Obvious? How? Do I go dressed in a sequined beach cover-up? Or was there such a thing as *Black Tie Swimwear*? Now that's a scary thought: Would I have to watch my fellow Jews dance the Hora in Gucci thong bikinis?

You have to give my daughter credit for trying to explain *Black Tie Beach Wear*, mentioning things like: beach bag type purse and dressy sandals for me while her father could wear an *I Love Venice Beach* T-shirt under his tuxedo. However my husband and I finally decided to wear our usual formal attire with one concession: we lathered ourselves with sunscreen. At least we smelled the part.

The ceremony, held at a yacht club, reflected the theme. The groom wore a tux made out of a bright Hawaiian print while the bride wore traditional white, if you call wearing a bikini under a see through white lace dress traditional. As a final touch, after being pronounced husband and wife, they stepped onto a surfboard fitted with tiny wheels and were pulled up the aisle into the reception hall laid out with tables, beach umbrellas and servers wearing beach cover-ups. "How festive," I thought, as we approached our table and sat down next to the only pair already seated.

I recognized one of the women as the bride's mother's housekeeper who had evidently come with a friend. "Hi Blanca," I said. "Do you remember us? Alice and Jesse?"

She smiled, nodded and said, "Hello."

"And your friend's name is …" I said, looking towards the other woman.

Blanca didn't answer, which seemed a bit odd, but the other woman finally said, "Josefina."

"Nice to meet you," I said. She nodded and smiled but didn't say anything else. Maybe I needed to break the ice, so I asked: "Did you watch the Academy Awards last week?" No response. Maybe she didn't hear me, so I repeated the question.

This time Blanca answered: "I'm fine."

Comprehension finally dawned. I leaned over and whispered to my husband, "I don't think they speak any English."

"I figured that out," he whispered back. "I guess we'll smile a lot and hope the food is good."

After what seemed like decades of smiling, another couple finally arrived. She was a tall, stunning blonde sporting a ponytail and a slinky black dress that just managed to cover a pair of expensive breasts. I couldn't help wondering what that black number would look like on me, but one glance down at my own shape and I put an end to that thought. Instead, I tried not to stare at her tall, handsome husband sporting tight, black pants and an even tighter T-shirt that revealed his bulging muscles. Unfortunately, I did not catch their names because I was too busy wondering if Mattel could market them as *Black Tie Beach Wear Barbie and Ken*. I was still pondering this when I heard Barbie ask Josefina and Blanca:

"How do you know the bride or groom?"

"I'm fine, thanks," said Blanca smiling.

"Me, too," said Josefina smiling.

Apparently Barbie had both looks and brains. She immediately grasped the situation and moved so she and her husband could sit down next to us. Ken gave me a friendly look before announcing:

"We are very close friends of the bride's family. Who are you?"

What an odd thing to say. It gave me an inane wish to answer: We're very close enemies of the bride's family. "Instead, I avoided the issue altogether by asking them both: "What did you think of the ceremony?"

Only Barbie answered. "It was fab-oo-luscious! How clever to pull the bride and groom down the aisle on a surfboard. And I loved the bridesmaids in their long, black sarong wraparound skirts and halter-tops. Although I have to say that I didn't care for the shorter sarongs on the groomsmen. Four pairs of hairy legs were a bit much. They should've shaved them. My husband always waxes his legs in summer. Does yours?"

Fortunately, I didn't have to answer that question since her cell phone rang. How she heard it in that din was beyond me. Yet the noise didn't affect her entering what I call "cell phone space." With Barbie occupied I turned to Ken and once again tried a conversation opener: "Did you see the Academy Awards last week?"

He nodded and smiled. Talk about deja vu. Was there something in the air? I tried again. "So, did you watch the Awards?"

At least this time I got an answer: a truly offended look. Not knowing what to do I kept quiet and waited for him to reply, which he finally did: "I don't have a Ford, I drive a BMW."

I was confused. Really confused. So I started babbling. "I didn't ask about your Ford. I said 'award' since the truth is I wouldn't know a Ford from a BMW if one hit me over the head. I drive a white Camry sedan and I often mistake other cars for it. Just the other day I was desperately trying to open the door of my car when a guy rushed out of a store to stop me from stealing his white Mercedes. He didn't seem to believe me when I told him that I thought his car was mine."

Yet Ken still didn't smile, laugh or answer me. It was Barbie who finally addressed my escalating bewilderment by leaning back in her chair so she could speak behind his back. "He's very hard of hearing. Even though he's wearing his hearing aids, it's too noisy in here for him to hear much."

"Oh," I said, turning a surprised look into one of sympathy. "Thanks for telling me. I'll try to speak a bit louder." However, I soon realized that Ken didn't need my verbal assistance since he had a distinct advantage in this noisy room. He had started waving his arms around evidently communicating with Barbie through American Sign Language. I was absolutely fascinated.

"I wish I knew what he was saying," I whispered to my husband, as Ken continued to move his arms around.

"What are you talking about?" asked my husband.

"I'm watching Ken sign!"

"Ken isn't signing, he's doing biceps curls."

"Are you sure?"

"Yes."

"But why?"

"I don't know why," said my husband. "Maybe that's how he entertains himself when he can't communicate in a crowd." My husband could be right. Every time Ken flexed his mammoth muscles a slight grin appeared on his face.

I began to wish that I could amuse myself so easily since Barbie, once again, was consumed by her cell phone. At some level I had to admire her. To be able to cell yell amidst the roar of the revelers went beyond any "call of duty." She had so perfected her cell scream that a number of people heard her make carpool arrangements for the coming week. She finished by asking the person to call her back. She then put her phone down in the center of the table and stared at it. She didn't talk. She didn't move. She just sat there, staring, which made me think of a better name for Mattel to market her as: *Cellular Barbie.*

So there I sat, smelling of sunscreen, with non-English speakers to my left, a deaf man on my right and a ringing phone in front of me. What to do? Should I try to remember some high school Spanish, gaze at a cell phone centerpiece or work out with a hearing impaired Richard Simmons? With such choices before me, I turned to my dearly beloved and whispered:

"I'm having a hard time."

"Me, too," he said. "This doesn't feel real."

"But I think I know how to get through it," I said. "Let's use the '*why don't we just pretend we're stuck in a Woody Allen movie trick.*' Then all these odd goings on will seem fine because we're just following a comic script."

"That'll work," he whispered back, "as long the hulk sitting next to you doesn't try to bench press the table in the next scene."

The arrival of a very normal looking couple gave me a chance to hope that our featured roles in the movie might end. However they sat down next to Josefina, never introduced themselves and didn't speak to any of us. They might have been silenced by the almost simultaneous arrival of the final duo, a couple that I had met before. While he is a quiet man, his wife is known as the "Meshuggeneh." For those of you who didn't attend schools with Yiddish bilingual education, meshuggeneh means someone who is daft or nuts. True to her nickname, the Meshuggeneh sat down next to Barbie, clasped her hands to her head and said:

"I have such a migraine headache. I hope I don't start throwing up."

"I hope so too," I said. Everyone else seemed too stunned to say anything.

"Don't get your hopes up," said the Meshuggeneh. "I have throbbing pain and wave after wave of nausea. I better start taking deep breaths. That might help."

She began to breathe deeply while I suggested in a gentle voice, "Maybe you ought to go home. I'm sure everyone will understand." I then looked toward her husband for support only to note an empty chair. He had conveniently fled.

"And miss a meal that cost so much money? What kind of a person would do that? I am going to sit here and eat it all even if every last bit of it comes right back up," said the Meshuggenneh.

Since I had no idea how to answer that, it was a relief to hear Barbie's cell ring. Her friend had called back to confirm carpool arrangements five days from now. She then replaced the phone on the table. This encouraged the Meshuggeneh to show off her sense of humor by saying, "I hope I don't throw up on it."

Fortunately, a momentary reprieve arrived in the form of the photographer. He artfully arranged us around one end of the table and prodded us to smile. That elicited a groan from the Meshuggeneh but at least she did manage not to clutch her tummy during the photo-op. So we all looked fairly normal proving just how deceptive a picture can be.

By the time we sat down again, a waiter arrived with our salads. Unfortunately, right as he reached over to place mine, Barbie's phone rang. He jumped. Lettuce went everywhere.

"I'll bring you another salad," he apologized.

"No problem," I said, helping him retrieve stray bits of radicchio and endive. I got so caught up trying to subtly remove a small cucumber slice that had slid down my neckline that I didn't immediately notice the two empty chairs and the untouched food. The silent husband and wife had fled. This didn't surprise me. Woody Allen movies are not for everyone.

The Meshuggeneh, however, had a different take on the disappearance. She turned to Barbie and declared, "Can you believe that couple left before the meal? Some people are so rude!"

Barbie agreed. "So many people today lack manners." She then reached for her phone to make another call.

I spent the rest of dinner in quiet conversation with my spouse mostly discussing one topic, how soon we could leave. "Forget dessert," I said. "As soon as we finish the salmon, that's our cue to leave."

"Did you say something to me? I didn't hear you," said the Meshuggeneh.

"I was just mentioning how moist the salmon is," I said.

"It is good. I just wish I could enjoy it more," she said, as she took a spoonful of sauce to lick. She then turned to Barbie to say, "Your husband sure is a quiet man."

"He's hard of hearing. He wears hearing aids in both ears."

"Really?" said the Meshuggeneh, in an astonished tone. "Can he hear us at all?"

"Maybe a little," said Barbie, "but it's difficult for him to hear anything when it's so noisy."

"Well, he really ought to learn how to read lips." Barbie did not reply but the Meshuggeneh paid no attention to this. She stood up, leaned across the table until her face was squarely in front of Ken's and yelled, "You really ought to learn how to read lips!"

I have no idea if he heard this or not, but I had heard enough. I turned to my husband and said, "I am going to the bathroom and I am not coming back …"

*   *   *   *

"Are you sure you weren't really stuck in a Woody Allen movie?" she asked. "That sounded like the real thing to me."

"As far as I know I was still in real life," said Dr. Alice, "and I didn't make any of it up. Not one bicep curl, cell ring or emesis threat. I can only be thankful that I remembered to pull the *let's pretend to be stuck in a Woody Allen movie trick* out of my beach bag. However, if you aren't familiar with Woody Allen you can pretend you are stuck in any movie or television show. You can even imagine you're part of a bad soap opera. What's important is pretending that you are just acting or reading a script because that is what diffuses the stressful situation. Once you start pretending you actually create a distance between yourself and the problem. This distance enables you to activate your Humor Antennae so you can start seeing the funny side of the circumstances."

"It's a clever idea or 'trick' as you call it," she said. "I might have to try it out someday. I might even pretend I'm a movie star."

"You can pretend anything you want," said Dr. Alice. "And you can have a lot of fun with this. I do, especially when I know ahead of time that I may be heading into an unavoidable but annoying or stressful circumstance, like having to spend a holiday with a family member who drives me nuts."

"And who doesn't have one of those?"

"And mine is so annoying," said Dr. Alice. "At a recent family gathering she spotted my grown son drinking wine with his cousins. This sighting inspired her to approach me with a sad smile and say: 'Alice, you didn't tell me that your son has a drinking problem.'"

"Wait," she said, "How does drinking wine at a gathering make one an alcoholic?"

"It doesn't, but she enjoys trying to cause trouble. She makes these kinds of comments all the time."

"Why?"

"I don't know and I really don't want to know," said Dr. Alice. "I only see her occasionally so it's easier just to go along with her agenda and I do this by using the *pretend to be in a movie trick*. This distances me from her zingers, saves me endless aggravation and gives me permission to have a conversation that doesn't make sense because I'm just following a script, right? And, it's fun to do this!"

"So what did you say to her that time?" she asked. "I'm so curious."

"I said with a completely straight face: 'Thanks for pointing out his drinking problem. I'll start looking for rehab programs as soon as I can. I've recently heard of a good one that uses prescription medication and chocolate bagels to spur recovery.'"

"That's funny, but in a sense, you did just agree with her."

"I did," said Dr. Alice. "I used a little humor for me and I agreed with her which was also important. The last thing I want is to escalate the situation. That would defeat the whole purpose of Coping Humor."

"I see that, but did she say anything about the chocolate bagels?"

"No. My guess is when she couldn't get a rise out of me she just moved on to her next target."

"I'll have to try that," she said. "I can think of a few relatives of my own who are not perfect company."

"You should give it a try. However, keep in mind that this trick works best when faced with everyday stress. I don't use this approach with deeply troubling circumstances or emotionally complex issues."

"You mentioned before that Coping Humor can help with complex issues, but isn't it difficult to use any kind of humor in those circumstances? Aren't there situations that no matter how you look at them are just not funny?"

"Of course there are," said Dr. Alice, "but that doesn't mean you can't use humor to brighten them. Patty Wooten, a nurse known for her work in bringing humor and humanity into the field of health care delivery, said it so well: *One can be open to the possibility that amusing events can occur even in the most challenging circumstances.*"

"I still find that hard to believe," she said.

"Maybe you'll better understand it if I tell you that Coping Humor takes a different approach under these circumstances. You don't look for humor in the situation because that might be impossible. Instead, you search for the humor situated outside the problem. And when you find it, you gently bring it forth to lighten up the troubling circumstance."

"That doesn't sound easy," she said.

"I'm not saying it's easy but you might be surprised at how much one can come to rely on this," said Dr. Alice. "And when it works, it can make a truly beautiful and memorable moment."

"It sounds like you're thinking about a specific moment, Dr. Alice."

"I am. I'm thinking about my friend Nancy who had a lovely life: an adoring husband, two nice boys in college and a job she enjoyed, but then she began to feel tired all the time. After seeing her doctor, my dear friend received the worst possible news."

She looked horrified. "Please don't tell me that she is going to die?"

"I did say it was the worst possible news."

"And you are going to find humor in this?"

"No, I am not going to find humor in the situation. That would be impossible," said Dr. Alice. "But I was able to find some humor for Nancy and for me because we needed it. However, if you don't want to hear about this, I'll stop."

"Please, go on."

"That wasn't all the bad news in Nancy's life. At the same time her husband was unfairly fired from his job, so he was without salary, health insurance and a recommendation for another job. He had to hire a lawyer. With so much going on in her life, I didn't tell Nancy that my husband had also come down with a serious illness. However, unlike Nancy, his prognosis was excellent. But she heard about him anyway and contacted me. I will never forget that phone call."

"What did she say?"

"She wanted to know if there was anything she could do for me."

"Are you serious?" she asked.

"I am."

"I don't know if I could've done that. What did you say?"

"All I remember is feeling overwhelmed by such a loving and giving thought when her life was so ..."

"Words can't really describe it, can they?"

"No, they can't," said Dr. Alice.

"When I think of all the little things I stress over," she said, "it makes me think we need another word for the tension created by these kinds of problems."

"What a good idea," said Dr. Alice. "How about super-sized stress?"

She tried not to smile, but failed. So she just shook her head saying: "I can't believe you said that."

"But my words did give you a break from the tension of the story, didn't they?" She nodded. "And all I did was make fun of a phrase, not the situation, right?" She nodded again. "So it's okay for you to smile. It really is. That's how humor works in these situations."

"I guess I can see that, but it's still something that may take getting used to."

"Of course, but the first step to using humor under difficult circumstances is to give it permission to enter the scene," said Dr. Alice.

"Okay, but it's such a new way of looking at things."

"But better, I hope."

"I'm considering it," she said, "but go on with the story."

"Things did get better. Her husband's lawyer settled out of court giving him a year's salary, health benefits and a recommendation that landed him a better job, although it meant moving two hundred miles away."

"How difficult for your friend. To have to leave family and friends when you have so little time."

"Actually, it worked out. Her family is all in England and she moved to a neighborhood where she was befriended by a close group of women who were just wonderful to her. However, she continued to decline and soon I knew I needed to go say good-by.

"How, how ..."

"It was so, so ... well, no words can describe how hard it is to say good-by to someone so special and loving. Anyway, I made arrangements to go see her. She was thrilled and said: 'I so hope that I will be having a good day when you come, Alice, because I want more than anything to laugh with you."

"Did that put pressure on you?"

"Actually, no, because it gave me something to concentrate on besides the reality of the situation. I drove down to spend the night with another friend who lives about 25 miles from her. Early the next morning Nancy called with good news."

"She was having a good day?"

"She said that she woke up feeling absolutely lovely and that she wanted to meet me at a small seaside town located between us. However, she did warn me about something."

"What?"

"'Alice,' she said, 'I do look a bit yellow.'"

"And what did you say?"

"The truth, that yellow is my favorite color," said Dr. Alice. "She not only laughed, she told me that she couldn't wait to see me because it would be so nice to be with someone who was not afraid to joke with her."

"So did you laugh together?"

"We laughed, we chatted, we shopped and soon, too soon, it was time to say good-by. For good. Nancy made it clear that she just wanted her family with her at the end. Talk about feeling emotional. I was feeling so emotional that it took me longer than usual to realize that Nancy was standing under one of my favorite street signs."

"You have a favorite street sign?"

"I keep a list of humorous street signs and I have my favorites. This one said: SPEED HUMP."

"Wait," she said to Dr. Alice, "Don't these signs usually say SPEED BUMP?"

"Not anymore," said Dr. Alice. "Now they usually say HUMP, which I find extremely funny."

"It is."

"So you, too, have heard the word 'hump" used as a slang term for an act that may lead to procreation."

She couldn't help smiling. "That is certainly the most elegant description of the term 'hump' I ever heard."

"Those are the exact words I used to explain the sign to Nancy. After all, I was speaking with a Proper English Lady."

"Did you point this sign out to her?"

"Of course I did," said Dr. Alice. "She was not that much of a Proper English Lady. I grabbed at that Humor Hook as if it were a life-line."

"And you both laughed?"

"I can still hear it. Being from England she didn't know the term, but as soon as I explained it she not only cracked up she asked: 'Alice, who is coming up with these signs?'"

"I don't know," I said to her, "but whoever he or she is, they are either not a native English speaker or they are having the time of their life with this. Either way, it comes down to this: we get to say good-by under a sign suggesting that we should be having a 'quickie.'"

"A Kodak moment," said Nancy, pulling a camera out of her purse and looking around. "I have to have a picture of this. Do you see anyone who could snap us under this brilliant sign?"

"Fortunately, at that moment a young man walked by who agreed to record this for posterity. As he raised the camera I whispered in Nancy's ear: 'Should we say cheese or shag?' That set her off again. She was still laughing as I drove off ..."

There was nothing for her to say as Dr. Alice's thoughts were, for the moment, hundreds of miles away. And that was okay because, she, too, needed some time to reflect. She had never spent much time thinking about using humor to relieve or deflect stress, although she had certainly tried enough other ways to relieve anxiety. She loved a good massage, but you couldn't use that in the middle of a stressful wedding or a final good-by. She had also tried yoga, but she had yet to figure out what made it relaxing. Twisting one's body into weird positions was not comfortable or comforting. Now, meditation was nice, if she didn't fall asleep, yet one couldn't use it in the moment.

The more she thought about Coping Humor, the more she realized how unique it was. You could use it alone or with others. It was always with you wherever you went. You didn't have to sign up for it, drive to it or make special time for it. And there was nothing to buy. You just had to buy into it. That was sounding more and more appealing because she couldn't think of anything else that could use something as absurd as Swedish meatballs to relieve anxiety before smoothly transitioning itself into something almost Shakespearean in nature. Didn't the story of Nancy show how 'laughter can make parting a sweeter sorrow?'"

"I'm so sorry," she heard a voice say. It was Dr. Alice returning from wherever.

"No problem," she said. "I, too, needed some time to think. Nancy's story gave me quite a new perspective on why I should be Humorized. Yet, I am still left wondering ..."

"About?"

"I guess what I want to say is that I would like to have more humor in my life and in some ways this seems easy. It will be fun to activate my Humor Antennae or just watch more funny DVD's."

"That's a great start," said Dr. Alice. "Just doing that will give you a physical and mental boost. And if that's all you ever do, that's great, too. However one feels comfortable using humor in their life is what they should do."

"Yes, but …"

"But what?"

"I would really like to use the Humor Hook. You make it sound so helpful and easy, yet …"

"Are you trying to say," said Dr. Alice, "that you want to use Coping Humor but you need a few more humor skills or techniques to feel comfortable with it?"

"I think I do."

"Then it's your lucky day. As a laugh doctor trying to start a Humor Revolution, I come armed with a Humor-Self Portrait, Laughing for the Joy of It and the Weapons of Laugh Instruction. All of these ideas can help you laugh more and stress less."

"Are you saying you run a laughter boot camp?"

"A laughter boot camp?" said Dr. Alice smiling. "That's quite an idea. I could call myself General Chuckle and run around yelling: 'You! Give me forty! Now! And make it laughs or giggles!' But I don't think it's necessary because all you really need to do is learn a few, simple techniques starting with the Humor Self-Portrait."

"A Humor Self-Portrait?" she asked. "I can't do that. I can't even draw stick figures."

"Neither can I!" said Dr. Alice. "If I had painted the Mona Lisa, it would have been called the Moaning Lisa. Fortunately, I'm not talking about art."

"Then what are you talking about?" she asked.

"I'm talking about an opportunity for you to just think about yourself."

"Really?"

"Yes, I am giving you permission to start chanting 'me, me, me!' Because a Humor-Self Portrait is all about you."

"I like that idea," she said.

"Most people do," said Dr. Alice. "Most people do."

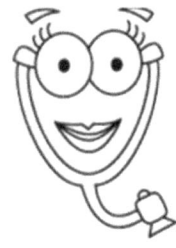

Laughing with Dr. Alice
Experience the Power of Joy

8. *The Humor Self-Portrait: Discover your Laughter IQ*

"Are you ready to start chanting me, me, me?" asked Dr. Alice.

"Not really," she said, "but you can to tell me what a Humor Self-Portrait is."

"A Humor Self-Portrait is a compilation of what makes you laugh and what makes you cringe."

"Is that all?" she asked.

"That's it," said Dr. Alice.

"So it's not one of those self-assessment tests to see how humorous I am?"

"Oh no," said Dr. Alice. "It's definitely not that because I am very uncomfortable with anything that rates or tests someone's 'humor abilities.'"

"Why?"

"What if I say to you, I've got this friend Linda who's just hilarious. She's one of the funniest people I know. Does that make you want to meet her?"

"Yes, I love funny people."

"You're not alone. Who doesn't enjoy being around people who make us laugh? We might even wish to be more like them, right?"

"Right."

"So, if I give you a humor self-assessment test and you don't 'do well,' how might you feel?" asked Dr. Alice.

"Bad."

"And who needs that feeling?"

"Not me."

"Not anyone," said Dr. Alice. "Because if you or anyone else develops negative feelings about humor, it defeats my whole purpose. My goal is for people to feel optimistic and relaxed, not uptight over a test result. So I created the Humor Self-Portrait. It's not a test, but a fun and insightful journey into your humor self to discover what tickles your funny bone and makes up your Laughter IQ."

"So Laughter IQ is not a number or an ability?"

"Absolutely not. Your Laughter IQ is just your own understanding of what makes you smile or laugh."

"And this differs from a Humor Self-Portrait …"

"Your portrait is a list of what makes you laugh and cringe which leads you to understanding your Laughter IQ."

"I get it, but …"

"But what?"

"If I discover more about my whole humor picture and Laughter IQ, won't that in itself improve my ability to enjoy and use humor?"

"It will, but without the worry or stress of testing!"

"That does sound a lot more appealing," she said.

"It is! It can also be exciting to look at a finished Humor Self-Portrait and think: This is what makes me laugh. This is my Humor Self. This is my Laughter IQ."

"So it really is all about me."

"It is because humor is very personal," said Dr. Alice. "What makes you smile may make another roll her eyes."

"That's so true. I often find my husband laughing at some joke that I think is just dumb or I find myself keeping quiet during a discussion of a popular sitcom that I find dull."

"And that's why the Humor Self-Portrait has a place for your Likes and for your Dislikes. With humor, there are no right or wrong choices there are only your choices. What you don't like is just as important as what you enjoy so it's okay not to like jokes or that hot new sitcom that everyone is talking about. Your Humor Self-Portrait is all about you, not what's hot on the humor market."

"I see that, however …"

"Yes?"

"It's still not always easy or comfortable to admit that you don't like what's hot on the humor market."

"I completely understand," said Dr. Alice. "And that's why I added one more category to the Humor Self-Portrait. I call it Dirty Little Secrets."

"Dirty Little Secrets?"

"I know what you're thinking," said Dr. Alice, "but in this case 'Dirty' has nothing do with being R-rated."

"I'm disappointed!"

"Sorry, I'm just a G-rated girl," said Dr. Alice. "That's why A Dirty Little Secret is nothing more than humor that you might like or dislike, but you're embarrassed about admitting it. Since everyone has some type of humor they feel uncomfortable sharing I added this category."

"So the Portrait has three categories?"

"Yes. Likes, Dislikes and Dirty Little Secrets make up the Humor Self-Portrait. But you can see for yourself what it looks like."

"Well," she said as she looked it over, "this certainly looks like more fun than a self-assessment test."

"I think it is. In fact, when I give a seminar people get such a kick out of creating their chart that I often have a hard time moving on to the next subject. And guess what they like talking about the most?"

"Their Dirty Little Secrets?"

"Yes! It's like opening a can of laughs. I start by revealing one of my Dirty Little Secrets and suddenly everyone wants to share one of theirs."

"And do I get to hear one of your Dirty Little Secrets, too?" she asked.

"Why not? I love watching the old Don Knott's movies. He was a funny, gentle and endearing comedian. Fortunately my husband also loves to watch him bumble around in his G-rated movies."

"Then why is it a Dirty Little Secret?"

"Because my kids are totally embarrassed to have parents who watch *The Apple Dumpling Gang* or *The Ghost and Mr. Chicken*. What would their friends think? We have strict instructions to only watch *Hot Lead and Cold Feet* or *How to Frame a Figg* in the privacy of our bedroom."

"Are those the real titles?"

"Of course!"

"They're hilarious," she said. "Actually, the whole situation is funny. Having to go 'undercover' to watch G-rated movies."

"And that's just one part of my Humor-Self Portrait," said Dr. Alice. "When I filled it out for the first time I ended up calling a doctor of psychology. After seeing what I wrote down, I appeared to be in dire need of a therapist for Therapeutic Humor!"

"What did you write down?"

"After writing Don Knotts under Dirty Little Secrets, I turned to Likes and wrote Richard Pryor."

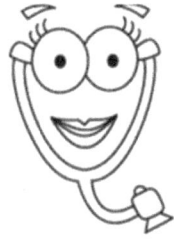

Laughing with Dr. Alice
Experience the Power of Joy

Humor Self-Portrait

Likes   **Dislikes**   **Dirty Little Secrets**

Directions: Under each heading list types of humor or specific people, movies, etc. such as: Stand-up, Slapstick, Wit/Wordplay, Cartoons, Farce, TV Sitcoms, Jokes, Funny Movies, Political Satire, Clowning, Favorite Comedians, British Humor, Comics plus anything you find funny!

She almost choked. "He is a bit different from Don Knotts!"

"Different doesn't begin to describe the difference. You have one mouthing four letter words as he rambles on about whores and drugs, while the other is the ultimate G rated comic. I looked at my chart and questioned my own sanity. Did I have a split personality? Or was I bipolar or schizophrenic? I called my friend Rick the psychologist and yelled, 'Help!'"

"And what did he say?"

"He said that my choices made perfect sense because both men used the same kind of humor. Was I ever relieved!"

"I would never have thought that," she said.

"I didn't either until he pointed out that both comics used self-deprecating humor."

"Self-deprecating humor?"

"When people make fun of themselves or of the situations they find themselves in, they are using self-deprecating humor," said Dr. Alice. "Both Richard Pryor and Don Knotts were masters of this. I'll never forget watching Richard Pryor frankly discuss catching himself on fire while he was free basing cocaine. He struck a match, waved it in front of the audience and asked: 'What's this?' His answer: 'Richard Pryor running down the street.' I still laugh every time I think of that line. Yet, Don Knotts constantly blundering his way through ridiculous situations also touches my funny bone."

"Dr. Alice?"

"Yes?"

"You described the Humor Self-Portrait as a simple list of what makes you laugh and what makes you cringe, but it's quite a bit more than that, isn't it?"

"Yes it is," said Dr. Alice. "It can lead you on a pretty amazing humor journey. Look what I learned from just listing two names on my Portrait. I now truly understand the type of humor that I love most. My funny stories certainly rely on my use of self-deprecating humor."

"You do like making fun of yourself," she said.

"I really do. In fact, I just finished writing one that totally uses my love of self-deprecating humor."

"And do I get to hear it?"

"If you aren't storied out," said Dr. Alice.

"Not at all," she said.

*   *   *   *

Another day. Another dinner. Another late afternoon spent roaming around the kitchen foraging for food. Why the empty shelves and barren freezer? Was it the drought? The lack of good soil in my kitchen floor? Slash and burn? Over-grazing? With such profound questions engaging my mind, I didn't pay much attention to my daughter who burst through the doorway yelling:

"There you are, Mom!"

I didn't react. I was too busy speculating if I could make a stir fry out of egg-plant, bananas and canned tuna.

"Mom, listen up. This really hot guy drove me home from school and he's here in the family room." I looked up at that. I may be over forty, but I am not dead.

"You want me to meet him?" I asked.

"No! I want to make sure you don't come near him."

"What?"

"Mom, I don't want this guy to see that I have a mom who looks like a bag lady."

Now, I admit that I don't exactly dress for success, and today was no excep-tion. I had on a pair of worn leggings, a UCLA Bruins sweatshirt so old that the only legible letters spelled 'ruins' and my hair hadn't been brushed since … but really, a bag lady?

"But won't he think it strange not to meet your mother?" I asked tentatively.

"Trust me. He will think it stranger if he does."

The young man in question did not stay long. After he left I judged it was time for my daughter and me to have a "heart to heart" or should I say, "looks to looks" talk. Why should she be ashamed of me? I was intelligent, loving and warm. What more could she ask for? I learned soon enough.

"You need to improve your appearance," she said.

"Being fashion conscious isn't everything."

"But Mom, you're in a fashion coma."

"I guess I could wear leggings without holes."

"I think you could do more than that," she said while a look of pure calcula-tion spread over her perfectly made-up face. I deemed it time to end this discus-sion quickly before she suggested the unsuggestable. Unfortunately, I was not quick enough.

"Mom!" I froze. She didn't.

"Tomorrow. You. Me. The Mall."

Now I realize that most mothers would be thrilled to have their teenage daughter ask them anywhere, and I would have love to go birding with her or watch an episode of *Antiques Roadshow* together. But the mall? Browsing? Shopping? Buying? Would I survive or would I fold under the pressure of trying to sneak four garments into a dressing room that only allows three?

The yell of "Mom!" momentarily jarred me from these terrifying thoughts. "Read my lips," said my daughter. "It's just the mall, not prison."

She had to repeat that statement the next day as she lured me out of the car and into an upscale department store. While I started breathing deeply, she went into her serious shopping mode, carefully scanning so many pants, tops and skirts that I finally drifted away only to notice that a sales girl had her eye on me. Now, the last thing I wanted was an encounter with some maniacal sales girl. I turned to flee from her when I saw another one approaching from the opposite direction. With no place to run I did the only thing possible. I dove into the clothing rack to wait it out. I have no idea how long I spent spelunking amidst ladies' pantsuits, however I finally heard a familiar voice.

"Mom, Mom, where are you?"

"Psst, down here," I whispered, poking my head out between a pair of red linen pants.

"Mom, what are you doing? You look like some red-eared rabbit."

"Hiding from the sales girls. They're stalking me. Are they crazy or what?"

"Mom, I don't think it's the sales girls who are crazy." She then grabbed my hand and led me into a dressing room. "Now, you are not to move. Stay. Do you understand?"

Not everyone likes being treated like a dog, but it worked for me. My only complaint about being cloistered in a fitting room was the lack of a nice lounge chair and a novel. Being a resourceful person, I decided to use the time to meditate. I sat down on the floor, crossed my legs and began to chant, "Oom ome nan, oom ome nan."

"Mom, what are you doing now?" hissed my daughter, as she entered laden with clothes.

"Meditating."

"Stop it at once. Everyone can hear you. I had to assure a sales girl that you are perfectly harmless. She was about to call security."

"Sorry."

"Just try on these clothes, okay?"

I obeyed and tried on clothes and clothes and more clothes. And as much as I might not like admitting it, I did end up buying several beautiful outfits. They were going to look great hanging in my closet. I was going to have to make a point of remembering to bring people into my bedroom to look at them.

"So, I guess we can go home now," I said to my daughter, as we went down the escalator and past the tuxedoed piano player now pounding out the song *Tradition*.

"Not yet, Mom."

"What do you mean, not yet?" I asked horrified. I felt like I had just climbed Mt. Everest only to find out that I had scaled the Matterhorn at Disneyland.

"You need new make-up."

"Maybe I do, but can't we do it another day?"

"Mom, your base does not match your skin, your powder does not match your base and your blush is so old that it has petrified." I couldn't disagree because I know virtually nothing about make-up. I was 34 years old before I even bought my first lipstick. While I would like to say that my late start was due to natural beauty, the truth is that it was due to natural laziness. Let's just say I couldn't be bothered trying to decide if I looked best in Paprika Peach or Pimply Pink.

At least today I wouldn't have to try to choose my own make-up. I could only follow the force marching towards a cosmetic counter that harbored a young man attired in black leather and sporting spiked hair, black eye shadow and purple lipstick.

"Hey, wait a minute," I said.

"What is it now, Mom?"

"You aren't planning to talk make-up with that guy?"

"Yes, I am."

"Why him? He looks like he ought to be selling war paint, not cosmetics."

"Mom, he is an incredible make-up artist. I have bought tons from him and he really knows his stuff."

"I don't know about this," I said, "I am not sure I want to buy make-up from some guy who looks like he belongs in *The Rocky Horror Picture Show*."

Before our disagreement could escalate further a reprieve arrived in the form of two of her best friends who screeched at the sight of her and then begged her to shop with them. I was happy to agree to give her up for an hour and headed off to the one place in the mall I loved: the bookstore.

Yet, even after buying my usual decaf single shot low-fat vanilla latte, I still couldn't stop thinking about my daughter and how fixated she is on "looks." It's not that she is an anomaly or anything. The truth is that her attitude is so common that the famous saying: *Beauty is in the eyes of the beholder*, works best as a slogan for the Braille Institute.

I have to think that General Lew Wallace, civil war hero and author of the above saying, would now agree with me because there is plenty of evidence to support my point. All I had to do was walk over to the periodicals and *voila*, there they were, dozens and dozens of magazines all devoted to making females more physically and sexually attractive to ourselves, to our men and to our dogs. Yes, I said dogs. One magazine featured a cover showing a woman wearing a zebra striped tank top and fringed jeans. On her lap sat a Chihuahua sporting a matching zebra striped vest surrounded by the words: *How to Make Yourself Irresistible to Your Canine Companion.*

I was about to put the magazine back when I noticed another article that grabbed my attention. It was called *Understanding the Secret Needs of your Lover's Scrotum.* The gist of the piece explained how the scrotum has always had an inferiority complex to another more anatomically exciting part. Thus the secret to being a great lover is to cheer up that "sad sack" by offering it equal respect and admiration.

That article gave me food for thought by raising a serious question: should I be paying less attention to migratory bird season and more to my husband's "sad sack?" Yet the scribe calling himself a "Scrotal Expert" never stated how one should go about doing this so I moved on to the next article, a regular feature offering advice on how to firm your body while performing everyday activities.

This month's installment was called: *Freeway Firmness or How to Tone Your Thighs While Going 65.* At least this writer clearly stated how to do it:

1. Merge onto the freeway.

2. To tone the right thigh, tense the upper leg muscle as your foot presses down on the gas pedal. Try not to suddenly accelerate.

3. To tone the left thigh, lift the entire leg up and down. To fully benefit from the exercise, use a rhythmic motion achieved by chanting, "Tense and lift, tense and lift."

Truly inspirational pictures accompanied the article, showing before and after shots of "women who drive with their thighs." And why shouldn't they? So many of us drive while drinking coffee, applying make-up and talking on the phone, why not exercise as well? Doesn't this make perfect sense? The article concluded by giving us the title of the next intriguing installment: *How to Have Abs of Steel While Eating a Fast Food Meal.*

I closed the magazine with my mind made up. There must be some value to making myself sexier and prettier. Why else have all these shelves and shelves of beauty magazines that offer thousands and thousands of beauty tips? Why not put more effort into being physically attractive to myself, to my man, and to my dog. Wait, I don't have a dog. Oh well, I'll just have to figure out how to make myself more alluring to my cats.

Believe it or not, all on my own I marched out of that store and headed to the make-up section in the department store. I bought some cosmetics from a very nice and helpful woman at a counter as far away as possible from *The Rocky Horror Picture Show*. I didn't tell my daughter. I wanted it to be a surprise. Already I was picturing her admiration and astonishment at my transformation: the new clothes, the make-up, the toned thighs and the abs of steel. Of course she wouldn't be able to appreciate my new insights into her father's scrotum, but you can't have everything.

In the end I was too impatient to wait for my new thighs or tummy to emerge. Just a few days after our trip to the mall, I clothed myself in one of my new outfits and applied my new make-up right before she arrived home from school. She walked in and behaved exactly as I had expected. Surprised. Speechless. Stupefied. Just when I thought that I had accomplished the impossible she began to laugh … and laugh … and laugh. Finally she stopped long enough to ask:

"Mom, why are you wearing lip liner on your eyes?"

$$*\qquad*\qquad*\qquad*$$

"Did you really put lip liner on your eyes?" she asked.

"I did."

"That's too funny. A make-up challenged doctor."

"But being make-up challenged doesn't bother me," said Dr. Alice.

"That's pretty obvious!"

"But it's also key to the humor in this story."

"How?" she asked.

"In this story, I let my audience know early on that appearance isn't important to me by clearly stating: *Why should my daughter be ashamed of me? I'm intelligent, loving and warm. What more can she ask for?* This attitude lets the reader know that since looks don't matter to me, it's okay to feel comfortable laughing at my cosmetic antics."

"You're right," she said. "I was totally comfortable with the humor."

"That's because you were laughing with me as I made fun of my behavioral quirks, not of myself. And that's why self-deprecating humor is a warm-hearted experience. This differentiates it from put-down humor that usually makes fun of who someone is and can be mean-spirited. It's important to understand this difference because put-down humor can make people uncomfortable while self-deprecating humor offers comfort and optimism. And I can't emphasize enough how important this is because as soon as a whiff of discomfort enters the scene, you lose the mirthful experience and all its amazing mind and body benefits."

"I guess that also explains why you have listed Dislikes on the Humor-Self Portrait," she said.

"Exactly. Humor has to feel comfortable and comforting which is why it's just as important to know what you don't like as well as what you enjoy."

"Dr. Alice, do you mind sharing one of your Dislikes? I admit to being curious."

"Sure. The first Dislike I put down was clowns. They make me very uncomfortable."

"Clowns? Why clowns?"

"Clowning feels forced to me, which is one reason I don't like it. But there might be more to my dislike. I had a rather traumatizing experience with a clown as a child."

"You were traumatized by a clown?" She tried not to giggle.

"Yes! I must have been about seven or eight when I went to the circus with a group. As you learned from my trip to the mall during the holiday season, I don't do well in huge, crowded areas. You can imagine how frightened I was when I found myself separated from my party and all alone until a clown appeared in front of me. I asked him to help me, but all he did was make funny faces that scared me even more. I finally ran from him and fortunately, found my friends."

"I think the clown meant well. He was only trying to cheer you up."

"Maybe, but that was not the right time or place for clowning around. Humor is not only very personal it also comes with a lot of sensitivity issues. Some hospitals today have clowns visit patients. Well, this wouldn't work for me! If a clown came to visit me in a hospital room, I might end up in intensive care."

She laughed then caught herself. "I guess I shouldn't laugh at that."

"That's okay," said Dr. Alice. "I meant to end the story on a funny note. But that's enough of my Likes and Dislikes. It's time to start thinking about your Humor Self-Portrait."

"Will you help me get started?"

"Are you asking me to become your personal humorizer?"

"A personal humorizer? That sounds so funny."

"It does make me sound like I unclog sinuses," said Dr. Alice. "So maybe I'll skip the title and instead ask you where you want to start, with Likes, Dislikes or Dirty Little Secrets?"

"Where do you think I should start?"

"Wherever you want. It's your portrait, remember?"

"But what do you think is best?"

"Listen, this is your self-portrait, no one else's," said Dr. Alice. "It's all about you, remember? So, why don't you just close your eyes, take a deep breath and just see what pops into your head. This is supposed to be relaxing and fun, remember?"

So she closed her eyes, took a deep breath and moments later a rather embarrassed, giggly look appeared on her face. Dr. Alice smiled and said: "I think a Dirty Little Secret just popped up."

"You're right. My favorite funny movie popped up, but I'm a bit embarrassed to say what it is."

"I shared mine."

"Okay, okay. It's Blazing Saddles, the Mel Brooks movie about a redneck western town that suddenly has to depend on a black sheriff to keep it safe from evil doers."

"It's one of my favorites, too!'

"It is?"

"Oh yes," said Dr Alice, "except of course for the beans and flatulence scene."

"Male humor!"

"Very male," said Dr. Alice, "but I love the rest of the film."

"Me too, but now I'm wondering why."

"Well, I don't need to call a psychologist to figure this out. Apparently, you like spoofs. A spoof relishes poking fun at the follies of the human race in a light-hearted manner."

"Blazing Saddles certainly does that!" she said. "I love the way the movie makes fun of so many of our prejudices. It's such a relief to be able to laugh at issues that we usually have to be so careful about. Yet, while the movie makes fun of our prejudices, I don't find it mean-spirited at all, do you?"

"No, because underneath all the silliness, it points out how absurd these prejudices are and how easy they are to overcome. In its own unique way, Blazing Saddles is both optimistic and hopeful."

"So maybe it's not such a Dirty Little Secret."

"It can be anything you want," said Dr. Alice. "What's important is to realize what you like. Can you think of something else?"

"I can. I love watching The Daily Show with Jon Stewart. And that's a spoof, too, isn't it?"

"Absolutely," said Dr. Alice. "Mr. Stewart and his 'fellow reporters' have a great time making fun of real news issues. And by just listing two spoofs you have discovered almost endless opportunities to amuse yourself."

"Well, that was easy."

"It is simple. Now the question is, can you figure out a Dislike as well?"

"I can because something immediately comes to mind: sitcoms."

"Situational comedies," said Dr. Alice. "That makes sense because they are nothing like spoofs. Sitcoms usually rely on jokes."

"And I don't care much for jokes," she said. "Mostly because I rarely get them. Just the other day someone told me this: 'A guy walks into a bar and guess what he says?'"

"I have no idea."

"He says, 'Ouch.'"

"Ouch?"

"Ha! You don't get it either!"

"No, I didn't," said Dr. Alice.

"What if I say, 'a guy walks into a bar as in a metal pole.' Do you get it now?"

"I do," said Dr. Alice. "But I don't find it funny."

"I don't find most jokes funny," she said. "They usually feel forced to me."

"Then sitcoms probably feel forced to you, too."

"They do and that can be difficult. People used to talk about Seinfeld as if it was the greatest thing on earth and I never found it funny. It made me feel so awkward."

"That sounds like another Dirty Little Secret," said Dr. Alice, "since secrets can be anything that you are uncomfortable sharing."

"So I would put Seinfeld under Dirty Little Secrets?"

"You could put it under Dislikes or Dirty Little Secrets or both. But remember, just because something is a 'hot item' on the humor market doesn't mean it's 'hot' for you and that's just fine. Really. Truly. Humor is not an 'in' thing. It's a personal preference. No one should ever judge or feel judged at what makes them or anyone else laugh. I may not like clowns, but I still want to encourage people who enjoy clowns to relish the experience. With that in mind, do you think you could fill out your Portrait?"

"I can," she said. "And I'll have fun, too, although I do think that humor is not as simple as it first appears, is it?"

"No, it's not," said Dr. Alice. "Humor is so many things. It can be simple or complex. It's very personal and comes with many sensitivity issues. And that's why there's now a movement in the field of Therapeutic Humor to bypass humor and go directly to laughter."

"Wait a second. Did you say bypass humor to get to laughter?"

"I did. Up to now, I have spoken of humor and laughter as an entity that comes together, i.e., humor causes laugher. However, this isn't always the case. Humor is an experience that can lead to laughter, but laughter can also be experienced without humor. The advantage to this is that while humor is personal and comes with all kinds of sensitivity issues, laughter is universal. That's why some people are enthusiastically embracing a concept called Laugh for No Reason."

"Did you say Laugh for No Reason?" she asked.

"I did, because I'm talking about laughing simply because you feel like a good laugh and that's why I call this Laugh for the Joy of It."

"That sounds rather odd, Dr. Alice."

"It may sound odd, but it doesn't feel odd. In fact, it feels absolutely wonderful."

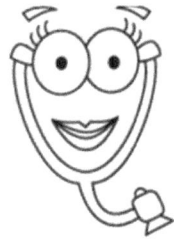

Laughing with Dr. Alice
Experience the Power of Joy

9. Laugh for the Joy of It

"I can see that you're a bit skeptical about being able to laugh for the joy of laughing," said Dr. Alice.

"How about more than a bit," she said. "Frankly, I find it hard to believe that it can work. It sounds so forced."

"If that's how it sounds then I can understand your skepticism, but I would never ask you to fake anything. However, if you agree, I would like you to try something fun that involves your whole body."

"My whole body?"

"Yes, I'd like you to lean forward in your chair, drop your head down towards your knees and dangle your arms," said Dr. Alice, demonstrating the position.

"Like this?" she said, as she slumped over.

"Perfect. Now, while you're still in this position, I want you to say: I'm so excited!"

She looked up and laughed. "I don't think that's going to work."

"Will you try it anyway?"

She agreed, slumping over once again as she said: "I'm so excited," in a voice that sounded less than enthused.

"I didn't sense much excitement," said Dr. Alice, shaking her head.

"That's because I can't convey excitement slumped over in a chair!"

"Then try this instead. Lean over again but this time I want you to suddenly jump up, throw your arms in the air and shout: 'I'm depressed!'"

"Come on," she said. "That's not going to work either."

"Will you try it anyway?"

"Okay, here it goes," she said, as she bent over before jumping up, flinging her arms in the air, and trying to shout: "I'm depressed." However all that came out was a half-choked giggle.

"Well," said Dr. Alice, "I guess jumping up and shouting didn't make you feel too depressed."

"Of course not. If anything, jumping up and shouting makes me feel energized."

"So your body action or your behavior actually generated a feeling?"

"It did."

"And did that feel fake?"

She paused before she said, "No."

"That's because body actions and nuances can and do generate true feelings," said Dr. Alice. "There is considerable research to back this up. One study showed that forced smiling enhanced the mood in study subjects.[30] Another had subjects voluntarily contract their facial muscles into various smiles, frowns and other expressions. The psychologists found that voluntary facial expressions generated matching feelings in the subjects. And this was not just a subjective test of answering questions. The researchers measured physical responses in the subjects' bodies.[31,32] This is an important point to consider. We take for granted that feelings lead to actions, like if you're feeling joyful you usually smile, right? But the reverse is equally true. We can smile for no reason and actually start feeling happier. However, I am not talking about just any kind of smile. I'm referring to a Duchenne smile."

"Duchenne?"

"A Duchenne smile involves the whole face, even crinkling the eyes. It's named after a French neurologist who mapped all 100 facial muscles in 1862. It used to be considered the 'real smile' that only happened after humor. However a study found out that even pasting a Duchenne smile on people's faces caused increased activity in an area of the brain responsible for many of our positive emotions.[33] It appears that this 'happy center' can be activated whether it's in response to humor or not."

"So you really can 'Put on a happy face?'"

"Yes and that's why I include this concept in the Humor Revolution. Would you like to try it?"

"You want me to force a smile and see if I start feeling happier?" she asked.

"Yes, but I don't like the word 'force,'" said Dr. Alice "Smiling is the start of a good feeling, so let's call it an intentional smile, okay?"

"Okay."

"So, are you ready to try it?"

"Not really. I feel kind of self-conscious."

"A lot of people say that," said Dr. Alice, "which is why I happen to have another high tech device with me."

"Not another snow globe?"

"Oh no, it's a straw."

She didn't know what to say that because it looked like an ordinary straw to her but maybe she was wrong. For all she knew it could sing and dance. Fortunately, Dr. Alice was not finished with her explanation:

"This is not just any straw. With most straws you put the narrow end in your mouth and suck, but not this one. When I put it in my mouth lengthwise, like this, I automatically make a Duchenne smile which can make me feel happier. This makes it such an incredibly special straw that I usually sell it for $500. However I can give you a special price. How about $300 for one or two for $500?"

"But wouldn't any straw do?" she asked.

Dr. Alice sighed. "That's what people always say which is probably why I never sell any."

"Do you try?"

"Every time I give a talk. I always offer my audience a chance to buy one of my special straws for only five hundred dollars."

"Do you really do that?" she asked laughing.

"I do, but my audience just laughs like you're doing. I have yet to sell a single straw."

"I'm not too surprised."

"And it's such a pity because my special straws could in handy in many situations like being stuck in traffic. Everyone knows how frustrating that is. But if you have one of my special straws in your car you can just stick it in your mouth and presto, you start feeling happier. And this makes other drivers happier, too. When they cruise by you and see you grinning and holding a straw in your mouth, they'll start smiling too. Talk about straw power. This little sucker can combat road rage and spread good cheer all at the same time. So don't you now agree that a mere five hundred dollars is a great bargain?"

"No."

"You're not the first to say that. Anyway, would you like to try putting a straw in your mouth?"

"No, thanks," she said.

"Why not?"

"Because I would feel like an idiot, Dr. Alice."

"I don't want that. Maybe you would feel more comfortable using an imaginary straw."

"An imaginary straw?"

"Yes, a straw no one can see. It can work just as well. When I'm in a stressful situation, I often put an imaginary straw in my mouth. While I'm not going to make any claims that it's a substitute for a true mirthful experience, it may help enhance your mood and that's not all. A study showed that it may jumpstart you towards a genuinely happy feeling." [32]

"And does this ever really work for you?"

"It sure worked at a birthday party I once attended."

"You needed one at a birthday party?" she asked.

"I did. I needed a straw and some clothes."

"Clothes? Why clothes?"

"Because …"

*   *   *   *

"What are you staring at, Mom?" asked my teenage daughter.

"An invitation," I said.

"To what?"

"My friend Jody's birthday party."

"That's cool," she said.

"It is nice that Jody is celebrating," I said, thinking that a birthday is the one time of year that our youth obsessed culture allows us to celebrate aging, "but I'm not too sure that I want to go."

"Why not?"

"It's being held at a naturist club."

"Did you say nature club?"

"No, I said natur-ist club."

"Is that, like, one of those nature centers where we used to go pet animals?"

"I guess you could call it a type of nature center," I said, "except there won't be any petting there since the only type of animal will be naked humans."

"Mom, you're kidding me, right?"

"I wish I were."

"Jody is having her party at a nudist colony?"

"She calls it a naturist club," I said, waving the invitation, "which is perhaps a good description since it must be an excellent place to study nature."

"I don't care what you call it Mom, old people partying naked is nasty."

How could I disagree? She had a point.

"You're not going to go, are you?" she asked.

"As a public health doctor it's not like I haven't seen naked people before. I guess I will have to think about it."

"Think about it? Mom, you don't even know how to dress stylishly. How are you ever going to pull off being fashionably naked?"

She had a point. So I decided to call Jody to kind of feel her out about the situation. "Jody, I'm calling to talk about the party," I said.

"Almost everyone has said they can come! I hope you're coming, too, Alice."

"I think so," I said. "I am still just a bit surprised by it all."

"Surprised? Don't you remember that I said I was going to have a really special birthday this year?"

"I just didn't think that special meant naked."

"Alice, are you uncomfortable with the nudity part?"

"Some parts of me are," I admitted.

"Forget about it. You are going to love the feel of fresh air on your nipples. Trust me. The club is absolutely beautiful and you will experience a connection with nature that is incredible."

"I will?"

"Besides, it's an all girl party and I am purposely having it on a Thursday afternoon since very few people go to the club on a week day. Does that help?"

"That does make it less, less …"

"And don't forget that the club is a clothing optional experience. I think that a birthday suit is perfect for my gathering, but if you really don't want to be naked, you don't have to be."

"How reassuring," I thought, as I hung up the phone. I now had the choice of deciding what would be less embarrassing: being nude in front of strangers or being dressed in front of nude strangers. After thinking about it for a day or so, I finally decided to throw caution and clothes to the wind and go. And, I was happy with my decision. Like most uptight, ordinary human beings I hate to think of myself as uptight and ordinary.

I do admit that I had second, third and even fourth thoughts about going. I even began to hope for rain in August, a month that could bring smog, fires, riots or an earthquake, but never rain. Oh well, why not pray for them all? Despite my best efforts, my prayers went unanswered. The big day arrived along with perfect weather for an outdoor party in the nude. I was never more frustrated. Even the Pacific Coast Highway, a road notorious for rockslides, sudden closures and horrible traffic, did not have one single slow down or tie-up. Where are SIG alerts when you need them? I even arrived at the club early and found my way to the "dressing room," clearly an oxymoron under the circumstances.

I might still be in that dressing room if I hadn't remembered the towel in my tote bag. Jody had mentioned swimming and I did not want to have to drip dry. I reached inside my tote and pulled out that large, blue piece of terry cloth that looked more beautiful than any priceless designer piece. After draping it around my body, I finally found the courage to venture out into the club.

It didn't take long to find my fellow party animals. They were all gathered around a large table covered with beautifully wrapped gifts. I sighed. How I wished I was as well wrapped. However, I did manage a smile and a kiss for the birthday girl; although for perfectly understandable reasons I chose to skip the hug.

She greeted me warmly. "Alice, I'm so glad you came. I know that you will just love being here."

I didn't reply because "loving the club" did not exactly describe my current sensations. It would be more accurate to say that I was so tense that if someone had hit with me a hammer, I would have shattered into hundreds of pieces all over the grass. Fortunately, Jody didn't seem to need an answer since she had already turned to the other party-goers to introduce me. She then proceeded to name people while I tried not to notice stretch marks, cellulite and such a garden variety of breasts that I was inspired to create the phrase: *No two boobs are alike, even on the same woman.* And while I did not pay much attention to the usual assortment of plums, pineapples and bananas, I did notice the bargain basement implant specials. I could only hope that if Jody ever talked about this woman in future conversations I wouldn't say:

"Oh yes, I remember Denise. She's your friend who has one nipple pointing up and the other pointing down."

My next move was to sit down, eat, and converse with my fellow guests. I did manage to sit and eat, but for unknown reasons my natural state seemed to cause an unnatural syndrome which I will call *body exposed, mouth closed.* Luckily, before Jody could notice the new quiet me, a diversion came along in the form of a stylishly dressed woman who strolled over with a camera and a copy of the club's monthly newsletter. She gave us a big welcome and said:

"I'm the editor of our newsletter and you ladies look like you are having so much fun! I want to know if I can take a couple of party pictures. You will make a great cover for our next newsletter."

"How exciting!" said Jody. "My party will be front page news!"

What was weird was that everyone but me seemed to love the idea. They started to arrange chairs, putting Jody in the middle, while I was wondering what I could do to make it through this moment without seeming like a party pooper. And that's when I remembered two things: my towel and my imaginary straw. I carefully reached down and draped my towel casually over parts of my body and then I mentally put that straw in my mouth as the Newsletter editor asked: "Are you ready, Ladies?"

She took her time taking the photo so I had that imaginary straw in my mouth for at least a couple of minutes. And what's funny is that by the time she left, I relaxed enough to finally see just how funny a birthday in the nude could be.

*   *   *   *

"I can't believe you went to a nudist colony," she said.

"Neither can I," said Dr. Alice, "but I have the proof."

"The photo?"

"Oh yes," said Dr. Alice. "Jody sent me a copy of the newsletter with our picture on the front cover."

"I don't think I could've handled that," she said.

"Actually it turned out fine."

"It did?"

"Yes, the photo was so blurred you couldn't identify anyone or see much of anything."

"What a relief for you," she said.

"It was a relief. I can safely say that I will never start a Naked Revolution. I would need more than a few straws to do that. However, on that particular day and at that particular moment, the imaginary straw really helped. It's a simple but fun thing to do but I don't think many people use it."

"I never have."

"Then maybe now is a good time for you to try it," said Dr. Alice.

"Now?"

"Would it help if I point out that you don't have to take off a single article of clothing."

"If that's the case," she said, "then maybe I will."

"Then before you change your mind," said Dr. Alice, "let's start smiling together."

The sight of Dr. Alice grinning as if her face would split made her, well, grin too.

"You did it! Now, isn't it easy?"

"It was easy, Dr. Alice, because your grin made me grin!"

"But that counts. You didn't smile in response to an emotion, did you?"

"No."

"And how did it feel?"

"Pretty good," she said.

"Are you less skeptical?"

"I am."

"Then maybe you're ready to try the next step, an intentional laugh."

"That sounds harder," she said.

"We'll start with an easy one called a smirk," said Dr. Alice.

"A smirk?"

"You smile while moving your eyebrows up and down like this."

"Dr. Alice, you look ridiculous," she said, chuckling and shaking her head.

"But at least I don't sound ridiculous. Now when I snicker ..." Dr. Alice grinned and snorted at the same time.

She cracked up. "Is that a snicker? You sound like a pig high on laughing gas."

"Do you want to try it?"

"No!"

"There are many other laughs to choose from like titters, chortles, cackles, guffaws, shrieks and belly laughs, to name just a few."

"A titter?"

"That's a high-pitched giggle," said Dr. Alice.

"And a chortle?"

"A supersized chuckle."

"And a cackle?"

"An energized, really loud laugh."

"And a guffaw?"

"That's a laugh that involves the whole body," said Dr. Alice. "Legs, arms and, as many of us can testify, the bladder."

She cracked up. "Oh my, change of underwear time? Just talking about this is too funny."

"But doing it is fun, too. Would you like to try a chortle?"

"That's the supersized chuckle?"

Dr. Alice nodded and began chortling and soon she couldn't help laughing, too, but not intentionally. So when Dr. Alice asked if it felt forced she had to say: "That's the odd part. It doesn't but that's because I soon as I hear you laugh or snicker I feel like doing it, too."

"That's because laughter is just plain contagious! You can catch a common cold and you can catch a common laugh. Just last week I was waiting in an airport lounge next to people jabbering away in a language I didn't understand, when suddenly they burst into laughter. Guess who couldn't help laughing even though I had no idea what was funny. And that is why it works. You may start with an intentional laugh but soon you end up laughing spontaneously."

"You really do," she admitted.

"Which is why Laughing for the Joy of It is such a valuable asset to a Humor Revolution. There is such a thin line between intentional and spontaneous laughter that ultimately both lead to Mirthful Laughter and its remarkable mental and physical effects. And laughing for no reason may also have an advantage over humor."

"What advantage?"

"We've seen that humor is very personal," said Dr. Alice. "Every Humor-Self Portrait is unique."

"No two Humor Self-Portraits are alike?"

"Exactly. Gather a group of people together, tell a joke and not everyone will laugh. Laughter is more universal because you don't need to get a pun or a punch line. Just start snickering or cackling and, before you know it, anyone watching or listening will join in. That's why a whole movement has emerged promoting the concept of organized laugh groups to the public. It began in India in 1995 when a physician, Dr. Madan Kataria, became concerned about the lack of joy in people's lives and how this could affect their health and wellbeing. He came up with an idea that began in a park."

"A park? Is this one of your diversions, Dr. Alice?"

"No! I am not making this up. In India people often walk together in public parks before going to work. Dr. Kataria thought that if people come together to walk, why not add humor too? He began by encouraging these walking groups to tell jokes, but this didn't work because humor is so personal and not everyone laughed. So he came up with another idea. Why not just laugh together for no reason at all? His idea worked so well he soon needed a name for these groups. He called it Laughter Yoga.[34] Today there are hundreds of Laughter Yoga groups in India and other parts of the world."

"That's quite a story," she said.

"And that's just one part of it," said Dr. Alice. "The popularity of this movement attracted the attention of a psychologist from Ohio, Steve Wilson. He went to India to study the idea and returned to the United States with his own spin on it, and with the help of his colleagues, started the World Laughter Tour, which encourages people to come together in Laughter Clubs to laugh for the joy of laughing. In the United Kingdom a psychologist, Robert Holden, founded Laughter Clinics that use Transcendental Chuckling, his name for simply laughing. People are literally Laughing for the Joy of It all over the world. And if you want, two more people can try it."

"You and me?"

"Yes, would you like to try a two person laughter group?"

"Is it different from what we just did?" she asked.

"Somewhat. A formal laughter group has a more organized format and is usually led by a trained laugh leader. Can you guess who might be one?"

"You?"

"I am a Certified Laugh Leader or CLL which means that I am qualified to lead a Laughter Club."

"Did you say Certified Laugh Leader?"

"I certainly didn't say certifiable," said Dr. Alice. "I was trained by Steve Wilson, the psychologist who heads The World Laughter Tour. We always begin with a warm-up." Dr Alice started clapping her hands and chanting: "Ho ho ha ha ha, ho ho ha ha ha."

The next thing she knew she was chanting and clapping with the doctor and feeling … well … rather playful.

"That's fun, isn't it?" asked Dr. Alice.

"It is."

"And that's just the warm-up before the first laugh which is usually a greeting laugh. I like to use the 'aloha greeting' but there's a twist. We are actually going to say a-lo-ha-ha-ha-ha-ha."

She managed to get out a few a-lo-ha-ha-ha-ha-ha's before she just cracked up. She then took a few deep breaths with the doctor before launching into a penguin laugh: walking around like the flightless bird while she tittered and chortled. And the laughs kept coming. Pretending to chat on a cell phone laugh, the eating spaghetti laugh and her favorite 'the gotta go' laugh. And in between each laugh, they took deep breaths and often repeated the warm-up: "Ho ho ha ha ha, ho ho ha ha ha."

When they finally finished she understood that laughter groups use hundreds of different kinds of intentional laughs that quickly morph into spontaneous laughter.

"I wonder if there is a group near me," she said.

"You can certainly look it up on-line. However if there isn't one close to you there are other ways to do this. I don't attend an organized laughter club, but I love simply laughing with my husband. I call him my laugh partner."

"Do you do this often?"

"We don't really have a set time, but it often starts as my husband comes home from work. He has a very high-powered job. Some days he comes home and I can just feel the tension in him. I used to greet him with: 'How are you?' but I think you know how he answered that."

"Oh yes. I'm sure he said: 'I'm all stressed out.'"

"So I decided we needed a change. I now greet him with a snicker or a titter or I may just run around him giggling and walking like a penguin. That always sets him off and we end up laughing together."

"Maybe I need a laugh partner," she said.

"Why not look around for one? He or she can be anyone: a good friend, a relative, even yourself."

"I can be my own laugh partner?"

"Why not? You can laugh all by yourself. There are a couple of ways to do this. You can sit and think about something funny or you can catch a common laugh on your own."

"I can laugh on my own?" she asked.

"Sure. Sometimes I like to sit by myself, close my eyes and giggle or chuckle just for the joy of it. You can do this too."

"I don't know if I could do that," she said.

"That's fine. While laughter may be more universal than humor, the appeal of Laughing for the Joy of It is still a personal choice. On a Humor Self-Portrait, it could be listed under Likes, Dislikes, or Dirty Little Secrets because someone might love it but be too embarrassed to admit it. While a Humor Self-Portrait is all about chanting, me me me, it's up you to decide if you want to also start chanting, hee hee hee! As I've said more than once, you need to choose the kind of humor and laughter you want in your life. Because if something doesn't work for you ..."

"... it won't enhance my mind and body," she finished.

"Precisely, so only you can decide if you want to include Laugh for the Joy of It in your life."

"It's something I will have to think about," she said. "Right now, after doing it with you, it sounds fun and appealing but, on the other hand, I am not sure if it's something that I will follow up on. It does have a silly side, doesn't it?"

"It does, but does that matter?" asked Dr. Alice. "Any new idea can seem silly or odd and this one is no exception. I have brought up behaving in a manner that up to now you may have thought of as childish or silly. You might want to reconsider this. Laughing for the joy of laughing is not childish, but childlike, which refers to behaving in a sweet and innocent way. As for silly, the word once meant blessed or happy. Maybe it's time to recapture that meaning because being silly in appropriate situations can be fun, relaxing and just plain wonderful."

"You sure seem to have fun with it," she said. "And your husband does, too."

"We do like it, but if you're not comfortable with it, there are other fun ways to increase the amount of humor and laughter in your life like using the Weapons of Laugh Instruction."

"And do I need a license to use these weapons?"

"Absolutely," said Dr. Alice. "Fortunately, I have with me your License to Giggle."

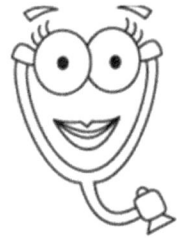

Laughing with Dr. Alice
Experience the Power of Joy

10. *The Weapons of Laugh Instruction*

"Dr. Alice, I can't wait to get 'Licensed to Giggle' but first, what exactly are the Weapons of Laugh Instruction? You still haven't really explained them."

"Then I'll jump right in by telling you that there are five Weapons of Laugh Instruction: The Truth, Exaggeration, Surprise, Irony and Parody. Each offers a unique way to develop more humor in your life. They are important and enjoyable tools for anyone wanting to join my Humor Revolution."

"And are they difficult to learn?"

"Not at all," said Dr. Alice.

"Really?"

"Yes, because I truly believe that most of us are naturally funny when given the chance. I sometimes host a 'dictionary party' where someone picks an unknown word from the dictionary. Everyone else then makes up a definition that is read out loud. I'm always amazed by the incredibly funny things people write. And sometimes the most hilarious definitions can come out of the quiet guy who rarely says a word. So I don't believe anyone has to take a giant step to add more humor to his or her life. What most people need is just to be gently reminded that they are innately humorous and should take advantage of this wonderful human trait."

"That makes me feel, well, warm and fuzzy," she said.

"It's supposed to," said Dr. Alice, "because The Humor Revolution should be a warm and fuzzy experience that leads us into thinking that we don't have to spend so much time running around as if you're over caffeinated and ..."

"... in need of a teddy bear to hug."

"You're becoming quite the comrade-in-laughter," said Dr. Alice, "which means that you're ready to hear about the five weapons. I think I'll begin with The Truth."

"Yes, do," she said, "because I don't understand it. How can The Truth be a technique?"

"It's not only a technique, it might be the most important one," said Dr. Alice. "Because even though we are innately funny, too many people allow too much humor to pass them by. I include The Truth to remind us of how important it is to stop, look and listen to all the humor that's right there in front of us."

"But isn't that the same thing as activating your Humor Antennae?" she asked.

"They go together," said Dr. Alice. "You need to activate your Humor Antennae so you can enjoy The Truth. If you think about it, this is what a stand-up comic often does. He or she understands that 'all the world's a comical stage' and to make you laugh, all they do is to point out the humor in a situation. But you don't need to be a comedian to embrace this technique. All you have to do is start looking for laughs in all the right places. Like the time I went to visit my brother in New England …"

✳   ✳   ✳   ✳

I was completely befuddled. Totally perplexed. Utterly baffled. And up to now, the trip had gone so well. I had left my toddlers with my husband in Los Angeles to luxuriate with adult relatives in the fall foliage of New England. After gaping at the kaleidoscope of red, orange and yellow surrounding Boston, I boarded a train to a small town in Connecticut to meet up with my little brother. But as I stood there waiting for him to arrive I felt like a living thesaurus of bewilderment because right in front of me was a street sign that said:

LIVE PARKING ONLY

What in the world was Live Parking? Did the town have problems with joyriding ghosts? Or were they worried that The National Association for the Advancement of Dead People, the NAADP, might want to hold a convention here? At least I had the perfect greeting for my brother when he pulled up:

"It's okay to park here, you're alive!"

"What are you talking about?" he asked, as I climbed into the car.

"That sign!" I said. "It's too funny."

"Funny? It's totally understandable."

"It is?"

"Yes, they are left over from when seafood vendors used to sell live lobsters at the entrance to the train station."

I was still contemplating on how live lobsters got translated into live parking as we arrived at scenic seaside town for lunch. Parking was tight so my brother was happy to find a spot in front of a house with an enormous front yard of solid concrete, every square inch of it. However, that didn't stop the owner from putting up a sign:

KEEP OFF THE GRASS

What could I do but laugh?

"What's so funny?" asked my brother.

"That sign," I said. "Do you see any grass?"

"No, but no one makes a sign: KEEP OFF THE CONCRETE."

"Maybe they should," I said, as we walked towards a restaurant right by a street sign saying:

DON'T PARK YOUR BOAT ON THE STREET

"Are parked boats a big problem?" I asked.

"They must be," said my brother. "Or why else have the sign?"

I was still considering this as we ate lunch and then headed down Interstate 95 to New Haven where we passed a large sign:

SLOW WHEN FLASHING

I couldn't help myself. I cracked up again. "What's so funny now?" he asked.

"That sign!" I said. "You never told me that flashing is such a popular past time in Connecticut. Is it more popular than joyriding ghosts or parking your boat on the street?"

He didn't laugh. He didn't even crack one smile. All he said was: "I can't believe how you read that sign."

"I can't believe the sign!" I said.

"You know that's not what they meant," he said.

"Maybe that's not what they meant," I said, "but you have to admit the wording is a bit questionable."

"I think it's fine," he said. I didn't want to get into an argument so I changed the subject as he parked his car alongside the curb in New Haven in front of a television repair shop. While he went to retrieve his TV, I waited in the car only to spot a street sign saying:

NO STANDING ANYTIME

How odd. Why aren't people allowed to stand there? Oh well, at least I was sitting, but two elderly ladies weren't. They were standing and chatting on the sidewalk with a cop car coming straight towards them. As a Good Samaritan I rolled down the window to yell:

"You two better stop standing there. You'll get a ticket!" The two ladies just stared at me like I was from outer space. Thinking they were hard of hearing I screamed even louder: "Hunker down! The cops are coming!"

My shrieking caused my brother to come running out of the store yelling: "What's going on?"

How was I supposed to know that NO STANDING referred to cars? Have you ever seen a car stand? "If they mean no stopping your car, why don't they just say so?" I asked.

My brother replied by saying that signs in Connecticut made perfect sense. "Just look at that one up ahead," he said as we merged back onto I-95 in front of a large, orange sign flashing the message:

WHEN RAINING WATER ON ROAD

What could I do but agree? That sign did make perfect sense.

*   *   *   *

"But that sign didn't last long," said Dr. Alice. After I returned home my brother called to tell me that the sign was changed to say:

WHEN RAINING ROAD MAY FLOOD

"How sad," she said.

"I thought so too," agreed Dr. Alice. "Why not enjoy a bit of fun while driving? We're always telling people to stop and smell the roses. Why not humor, too?"

"Except telling people to stop and smell the humor isn't going to fly, Dr. Alice."

"No, it's not even going to hover. And that's why I tell people to stop and savor the humor that's around them. And when the plain old truth isn't amusing, it can often be tweaked or embellished which brings us to weapon number two: Exaggeration."

"That one I understand," she said.

"While Exaggeration is usually apparent, it's still best to carefully consider a couple of aspects when using it. First, stick to universal or common subjects, because if you can't relate to the situation in the first place, embellishing it won't make it any funnier. It's also important to never over exaggerate. You have to be able to see some truth in a situation or the comical version won't be amusing. But when it all comes together, it can transform reality into something truly amusing ..."

*   *   *   *

It was a twelve-hour flight from Los Angeles to London. All I wanted was a quiet place to sit, snack and rest before taking my connecting flight to my final destination. What I got instead was London's Heathrow Airport. I can only suppose that two demented English architects once had the following conversation:

Architect #1: Do you know old top, I have come up with a simply smashing idea.

Architect #2: I could use a good upper, old egg. I have been feeling a trifle low.

A#1: I have an idea that will knock your socks off. So keep your pecker up, old chap, and listen.

A#2: I am all ears, you old goof.

A#1: I plan to design a new airport and I want you to assist me.

A#2: Right ho! That sounds like a dashed good idea, old chum.

A#1: Doesn't it? What is really dashing about it is that it won't be like other airports. I want to build a piping hot one by making the terminals several kilometers long and then, to make it extra smashing, make these terminals really far apart from each other.

A#2: But why do that, you daft old cow?

A#1: Just think what eye-popping fun that will be for the tired traveler.

A#2:. Start ho! Eye-popping fun indeed! Why you old stinker, you have hit on a really topping idea. I love the idea of designing a pear-shaped airport where people can fanny about.

A#1: Exactly, old chap. And to make our airport even jollier we can make the terminals so bloody far apart that people will need to take buses through long dark tunnels to travel between them.

A#1: What ho, old boots! Quite the idea! People will love waggling about in dark tunnels, what?

A#2: And that isn't my only idea, what? Let's fill those kilometer long terminals with posh shops, like Harrods. After people have walked for hours past hundreds and hundreds of shops they will be so barmy they will buy anything!

A#1: You are brilliant, old crumb. People will jolly well fancy that. But what about food, what?

A#2: What about it, what?

A#1: Do we need places where people can eat?

A#2: No, of course not, you silly ass. We're British, stiff upper lip and all that. We don't need food. Besides, everyone knows that the food in England is beastly. So why bother to serve any?

A#2: You're right about that, you old spindle shanks. However, I do think that after four or five kilometers of shops we could have a coffee house. You know the kind that those Americans love to potter around in.

A#1: Right oh, you old wanker. I know just the kind you mean, a place where those daft Yanks like to spend half their savings buying a cup of coffee with a fancy name. I think in America they're called some loopy name like Starducks.

A#2: Quack, quack, shift ho, is it all settled then you old ball whacker? Shall we start?

A#1: Absolutely, you old tottle head. I can't wait to create an airport so perfect that no one will ever call the British potty again.

$$* \qquad * \qquad * \qquad *$$

"Dr. Alice, I've had to connect at Heathrow Airport and what you described is not that far from the truth."

"And that's why it made you smile. I didn't have to exaggerate all that much. Heathrow does have long shop-filled walkways with few food options and at the time I thought of this, one did have to travel down, down, down to get on a bus and ride through tunnels to reach other terminals. However, since most people I know have had more than one frustrating experience at an airport, anyone can enjoy it."

"I also loved the wordplay," she said. "Apparently you are fluent in British speak."

"That's because I have devoured the books of PG Wodehouse, a prolific and hilarious English author who lived to be ninety-three," said Dr. Alice. "But I didn't have to exaggerate that much. I was recently at a family wedding where we all missed seeing a thirteen-year-old male relative who was in the hospital."

"Is he okay now?" she asked.

"Much better, thanks," said Dr. Alice." Anyway, another cousin bought an over-sized get well card and we all signed it including her British boyfriend who wrote: *Keep your pecker up, old chap!*"

"He didn't?"

"He did! To him, this only means keep your spirits up."

"Did you send it?" she asked.

"After a bit of discussion, off it went. The boy was thirteen, not three."

"And I'm sure he had a good laugh."

"And a nice surprise," said Dr. Alice, "which brings us to the third weapon."

"Surprise?"

"Does that astonish you?" asked Dr. Alice.

"No," she said, "because I love surprises."

"Most people do because a moment that's funny and surprising can really give you a jolt of joy that's an exhilarating feeling. So it's always good to be on the lookout for surprise even if it's often dependent on the right circumstances coming together."

"So it's a little trickier to manage?"

"It can be," said Dr. Alice, "but if a teen-age girl confined to a wheelchair can use it, I think other people can, too."

"A teen in a wheelchair?"

"Yes, she's been my daughter's best friend since middle school and is currently finishing up her bachelor's degree from one of the Pomona colleges. She was born with a muscle disease that has kept her in a wheelchair since she was seven. The good news is that her disease is not fatal."

"This still doesn't sound like an opening for humor," she said.

"Don't forget that humor surfaces even in the most challenging of circumstances," said Dr. Alice. "And Lexy is a funny, smart and insightful person who uses a wheelchair and a lot of humor to get through life. After you hear the story of the girls' first outing nine years ago, I think you'll not only see how special Lexy is you'll also understand how well Surprise works. And since my daughter wrote down what happened, you can hear it from her perspective ..."

*   *   *   *

"So this girl Alexis calls and asks me if I want to go to the movies with her. I said, 'Yes,' but I was a bit anxious because, well, I had never been out with someone in a wheelchair before. I knew she was nice and all that, and we were partners in English class, but still it wasn't going to be like going out with my other friends, was it? At least at that time I didn't know that we had picked like the worst movie ever to see. Anyway, her mom picks me up on a Saturday and drops us off at one of those large theater complexes. It's crowded and people stare at us, which I'm not used too. Anyway, we go to the concession stand because Lexy has to have a coke because she is like a coke addict. So she buys this huge drink and puts it by the side of her seat in her electric wheelchair and then turns around, too quickly. The coke goes flying, like everywhere and makes a big mess on the floor of the lobby. I am like totally embarrassed because all these people are staring. I don't know what to do or where to look, when suddenly, Lexy points at me and yells: 'She did it!' I started laughing really hard and so did everyone else. When I finally stopped, I realized something: I wasn't embarrassed anymore."

*   *   *   *

"How old was Lexy when this happened?" she asked.

"Thirteen."

"Amazing," she said.

"Lexy's really quick on her feet especially for someone who can't even walk. And her ability to use Coping Humor never ceases to amaze me."

"That story is certainly a great example of Coping Humor and Surprise," she said. "But isn't it also The Truth?"

"It is," said Dr. Alice, "because humor often relies on more than one technique. This story also includes the fourth weapon: Irony."

"Irony? I don't know if I see that but maybe that's because I'm not 100% sure I could define irony."

"It's the difference between the way we expect things to be and how they really are. This disparity can lend humor to a situation. The last person we expect to Humorize an embarrassing situation is Alexis, because in the minds of most people, she is the poor little girl in the wheelchair."

"I sure didn't expect her to lighten things up!"

"Who would? And that's what makes it ironic. However, irony can be trickier to see than other humor elements. This means that some people may not be able to find amusement in an ironic situation. My marriage turned into an ironic experience because it wasn't what anyone expected a wedding to be. Some people find the story terribly funny, while others find it just terrible."

"And am I going to be able to make that choice?" she asked.

"You are but first you have to know that my husband and I were once lovers torn apart by war, famine and the melting of polar ice caps."

"Are you sure about that, Dr. Alice?"

"Maybe the truth is a bit less dramatic. My husband and I were torn apart, since I was not accepted into medical school at UCLA where he was a surgical resident. So off I went to school in Atlanta. Fortunately, I had the option of transferring to

UCLA for my last two years citing our engagement, but I heard nothing for weeks. However, UCLA finally contacted my fiancé who called me with some startling news:

*   *   *   *

"UCLA says we have to show them a marriage license before they will accept you," he said. "Too many people fake an engagement just to transfer." He then casually added that we had two weeks to do this.

"Two weeks?" I said.

"We can do it," he said. "You fly home this weekend and we can be married at the Los Angeles County Courthouse on Monday. I've been given the morning off."

"Will that work?" I asked.

"No problem," he said. "They marry twenty couples a day during the judge's lunch hour. We'll be out of there by one."

"How romantic," I said.

"But there's a catch," he said. "It's first come, first serve, so we need to arrive early to make sure we're one of the lucky twenty."

Six days later we parked at the courthouse at 8:30 A.M. Ten minutes later found us standing at the sign-in desk manned by a figure sporting the largest blond Afro I had ever seen. All I could see of her face was half of one eye and part of a mouth. I was still wondering if she had some Picasso fetish as I heard her ask us to fill out the paper work and pay the $8.50 fee. My guy handed her a credit card.

"Sorry we don't take credit cards," said half-a-face.

I turned expectantly to my soon to be spouse expecting him to whip out the money but all I got was: "Do you have any cash?"

"Maybe three dollars," I said.

"All I have is two," he said.

"I can see that you two came prepared, but don't panic. I'll hold your place as couple #11 until the bank next door opens at 10," said the clerk since there were no ATM's back then.

"Thanks," I said, thinking that a Picasso face never looked better while my guy whipped out the parking ticket and asked for a validation.

"We don't validate," she said.

"You don't take credit cards and you don't validate?" he said. "What kind of courthouse is this?"

I laughed as if he was joking and then quickly dragged him away. "Paying for parking is a small price to pay for being couple #11," I hissed.

"I think this place needs to get with the program," he said.

"Our program right now is to wait for the bank to open," I said. So we did and soon paid up. All that was then left to do was wait for the judge to show up during his lunch hour. We passed the time checking out the other nineteen couples that ranged from people you wouldn't want to meet in a dark alley even if it wasn't dark, to a young, beautiful bride wearing an enormous white wedding dress accompanied by six bridesmaids clad in matching pink chiffon. At 11:45 A. M., the clerk finally made the announcement we had all been waiting for:

"The judge is arriving. All couples line up in numerical order with men on the left, women on the right, witnesses off to the side and no chewing gum!"

I choked with laughter. Whatever I had expected my wedding to be it didn't include being told to line up and not chew gum. I was still giggling as we entered the chamber at 12:30 for our three-minute ceremony. Since we didn't bring a witness, half-a-face stepped up to act for us asking: "Do you have the rings ready?" And that's when we looked at each other and realized that in the rush to be married, we had totally forgotten about rings.

"You forgot your rings?" she asked.

"No," said my almost husband. "We completely forgot about getting any in the first place."

"So, you came here without money and without rings to be married? You two are really well-matched," she said, as the judge started laughing. He continued to chuckle throughout the ceremony that, without rings, lasted an entire minute and a half. And while he didn't end with: 'You may now kiss your bride,' half-a-face did put in her two cents. She looked at us both, smiled and said: 'Well, kids, now you can go home and do it legally.'"

*   *   *   *

"Did she really say that in front of the judge?"

"Those were her exact words."

"Were you offended?"

"Not at all. We all laughed including the judge. And while I know this may be hard for some to believe, I wouldn't trade my crazy marriage for any number of fancy weddings. My husband and I still get a kick out of that day except of course, for the part about not validating parking. That still bothers him."

"And did you ever do anything else?" she asked.

"We had a great party several months later."

"Then it all worked out for you."

"It did. UCLA accepted me and we're still married."

"But I do have a question," she said. "Isn't this more parody than irony?"

"No, it's not but I'm glad that you asked that because irony is often confused with parody and they are very different. While irony is a discrepancy between what is expected and what happens, a parody deliberately copies other material, infusing it with a comic touch. And my wedding was certainly not based on anything that had happened before."

"So a parody is very specific?"

"Very and it's also the fifth and final Weapon of Laugh Instruction. And when it's done well, it can be so much fun."

"And if it's not done well?" she asked.

"It can not only be humorless, it can also be malicious. When using parody you have to careful to just make gentle fun of something."

"Keep it mirthful?"

"Yes," said Dr. Alice. "Do you know the book *Angela's Ashes*?"

"Of course. The best-seller and Pulitzer Prize winning memoir by Frank McCourt, but I wouldn't call it a mirthful read."

"No," said Dr. Alice, "Unless ..."

*   *   *   *

"Why are you working so late?" asked my daughter as she came into my home office at 10 P.M. "You and dad are usually a couple of zombies by now."

"I'm just too excited to sleep," I said.

"Why?"

"I'm writing my memoir."

"Your memoir? Why?"

"I've been looking around for a new creative project when I came across an article called *Write Your Own Memoir, Everyone Else Is*. What a great idea. I already have the two basic requirements needed to jump on the memoir bandwagon: a childhood and a memory. And I hear it's a great way to strike literary oil."

"But, Mom, who is going to want to read about your childhood? It was so ordinary."

"But the whole point of a memoir is to take an ordinary life and make it appear extraordinary," I said.

"Does that mean that you are going to tell a lot of lies?"

"No, I just need to figure out a way to make my childhood appealing and fascinating."

"That'll keep you busy," she said as she walked out the door.

Apparently I was going to have to search elsewhere for inspiration. At least I knew where to look. I scanned my bookshelves looking for *Angela's Ashes*. I loved this story because the author didn't just describe his life; he invited the reader to experience the deep aches and pains of growing up poor, starving and Catholic in a small Irish town. By doing so Mr. McCourt turned young Frank into a heroic figure and a much older Frank into a rich man. The book was on the New York Times Bestseller List for years, won the Pulitzer Prize, and had been made into a major movie. It also generated a best-selling sequel called *'Tis*.

It didn't take me long to locate the book and re-read the magic of its opening lines. However, this time I was more than captivated by the words. I was absolutely flabbergasted by the realization that there were similarities between Frank's cold and oh-so-hungry childhood, and my own warm and oh-so-haute cuisine one.

Now, I recognize that at first glance any parallels between a well-fed girl growing up in the wealthy and now infamous suburb of Brentwood in Los Angeles and a boy practically starving to death in Limerick, Ireland, may seem ridiculous. However, you may want to think again as you read, or as the case may be, re-read the opening lines from *Angela's Ashes*:

"When I look back on my childhood, I wonder how I survived at all. It was of course, a miserable childhood. A happy childhood is hardly worth your while. Worse than your ordinary, miserable childhood is the miserable Irish childhood and worse yet, is the miserable, Irish Catholic childhood."

Now, read how my story opens:

When I look back on my childhood, I wonder how I survived all that food. It was of course, a gourmet childhood. A fast food childhood is hardly worth your while. Worse than your ordinary, gourmet childhood is the gourmet American childhood, and worse yet, is the gourmet, American Jewish childhood.

I was amazed by how few words had to changed to fit my story. I yelled for my daughter who returned looking less than enthusiastic.

"Mom, what is it now? I'm trying to decide what to wear to school tomorrow."

"Read this," I said, pointing to the screen. I knew she would understand, because she, too, had loved *Angela's Ashes*. However, for some odd reason she did not get excited. Instead she asked:

"Is this some kind of joke?"

"A joke? How could it be a joke to discover that my childhood was just as riveting as Frank's?"

"Okay, Mom, forget I said joke. Instead, tell me why you are writing a parody of *Angela's Ashes*."

"I am not writing a parody. I am writing my own story!"

"Using Frank McCourt's words! Mom, it's a parody!"

"So, I'll change the words around," I said, as a new thought came to me. I, too, could name my memoir after my mother, just like Mr. McCourt did. He called his book *Angela's Ashes* because his mom, Angela, spent so much time smoking cigarettes in front of a cold, barren fireplace, which I believe, was a metaphor for their life. And while my mother never spent hours in front of an empty fireplace smoking Irish fags, she did have her own private agony, her excessive weight. She would spend hours going from her downstairs refrigerator to her upstairs one, from her outdoor freezer to her indoor one, gazing longingly at those white, forbidding ice-box doors knowing that they were packed with succulent delicacies that she shouldn't eat. What better way to immortalize her misery than to name my story *Naomi's Cellulite?*.

"Mom? Are you listening to me?" Evidently my daughter was still in the room.

"I am," I managed to answer.

"Then do me a favor. Before you write anymore look up the word parody."

So I did and realized my daughter was right ending my only attempt at writing the memoirs of a gourmet, American Jewish childhood.

*   *   *   *

"So you never did write Naomi's Cellulite?" she asked.

"No, I didn't," said Dr. Alice, "but I did share the little I wrote with my writer's group. They loved it even saying they wished Frank McCourt could hear it, but he has yet to contact me. That doesn't surprise me since it's not easy to talk to someone if you don't know they exist."

"And did you try writing any other parodies?" she asked.

"A few, but I'm most comfortable using The Truth. I've found that works best for me, and of course, you have to find out what works best for you. Think of the Weapons of Laugh Instruction as a buffet to choose from."

"Is it all you can eat?" she asked.

"It's all you can laugh," said Dr. Alice, "especially since there is more on this buffet than just humor techniques. There are all the mind and body benefits, the Humor Self-Portrait and the Humor Hook to name just a few. And you get to pick what you want to try."

"If I can remember it all," she said.

"Don't worry about all the details," said Dr. Alice, "because what's really important is to understand that humor and laughter need to become an important part of your life because they do amazing things for your mind, body and stress levels. They are a 'lifestyle treat' not to be missed since they will make you healthier and happier. However, I do have something to help you remember what we've discussed. It's called: The Humor Revolution: It's As Easy As ABC."

"Is it an A to Z list of Therapeutic Humor?" she asked.

"Fortunately for you and everyone else, I only got as far as E."

"That is a relief."

"And, to make it more of a relief, I've summarized the Humor Revolution into five ideas written as *Prescriptions*. Consider them remedies from a laugh doctor to help you stop inhaling stress and start inhaling humor. But you are going to have to look them over on your own time, because it's time for me to go."

"Right now?"

"Yes, but don't worry," said Dr. Alice. You still have Prescriptions A, B, C, D and E to help you Humorize your life."

"That sounds like a title from a Dr. Seuss book!"

"What a compliment. I love Dr. Seuss. Horton Hatches the Egg is one of my favorite books. I even have it on my Humor Self-Portrait."

"Really? I've always thought of him as just for children."

"I'm so glad you said that," said Dr. Alice. "What a perfect way to end our little talk."

"Little?"

"Maybe it wasn't so 'little' because now you know that humor is anywhere and everywhere: it can flourish in an airplane lavatory 33,000 feet in the air or in a display of singing Santa Claus underwear at a mall. It can lurk in a small town harboring odd street signs or in a furniture store the size of Florida. It can spring from a child in a wheelchair or from a children's movie about a ghost and a chicken. You may come across it at the wedding you never dreamed of having or with the friend you never dreamed of losing. So go forth and begin your own Humor Revolution! It can only make your life better."

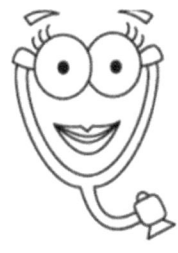

Laughing with Dr. Alice
Experience the Power of Joy

11. The Humor Revolution: It's as Easy as ABC

She was still in a sound sleep when her cat jumped on her jarring her awake. "When will I learn to close the door," she thought as she sat up to slide her feet into her now favorite slippers made of sustainable sheepskin and recycled pizza boxes. She then pitter pattered into the kitchen thinking she should start the day with a healthy breakfast.

Of course some people might think that a bowel of *Fiberlicious* cereal was healthier than the chocolate croissant she consumed but doesn't chocolate have anti-something in it? That makes it healthy, right? And she did plan to pop a few fish oils, too, except that she couldn't get the top off the container. She could've tried a bit harder, but she didn't want to hurt her hand and besides, wouldn't it be nice to step on a scale without anything extra in her stomach? She would weigh less, wouldn't she? Wait. Her scale was still broken. So she decided to return to her bedroom to slip into her new jogging shoes that were still in the shoebox. But then she might have to go outside and actually jog in the bitter cold of Los Angeles. Forget that. Instead she put on her hand woven organic cotton work out clothes with natural dyes but they itched so much she decided that she would skip working out on her exercise machine called *The Rack*. She didn't feel like pumping iron and itching at the same time. And besides, she didn't need to work out every morning, did she? Every couple of days was fine. Okay, so maybe she didn't work out every few days, but every week. Well, maybe once a month was more like it or actually every couple of months. And didn't she work out just last month? So she didn't really need to do it today, did she? There must be something else she could do instead to enhance her health.

And that's when she remembered Dr. Alice and her Humor Revolution. Hadn't the laugh doctor given her five prescriptions to look over? Where had she put them? She hoped she hadn't put them in a safe place. If she had, they were probably lost forever. Luckily, she soon found them piled on the kitchen table with 100 other piles of whatever. Of course, she did plan to organize her stuff as soon as The Pile Fairy appeared to help.

With the prescriptions found, she decided to make a nice cup of tea while she relaxed and read them. But first she needed to choose the tea: black, white, green, red or herbal? After several minutes of deliberation, she finally picked red roiboos tea infused with vanilla bean and cardamom. With cup in hand, she pitter pattered back to her bedroom, sat down and began to read:

The Humor Revolution: It's as Easy as ABC

By the time you look at this you have probably already heard me drone on and on for what seemed like forever about the benefits of humor on your mind and body. To help you remember some of the more important points I offer five simple prescriptions. Think of these as a remedy from a laugh doctor to help you stop inhaling stress and start inhaling humor.

Prescription A: All About You!
Get Ready to Chant: Me! Me! Me!

Humor is very, very personal which means that it's all about you! Isn't that a lovely thought? Don't we all wish that more of life was all about us! But with humor this is true. So ask yourself, do you cackle at stand-up humor? Jokes? Sitcoms? Cartoons? Political Satire? Or are you one of those that love to watch the same funny movie over and over again?

Understanding what makes you laugh and what makes you cringe is so essential I created The Humor Self-Portrait, a tool to help you figure out what activates your Humor Antennae so you can tune in Humorvision. In other words, it's a simple way to discover what kind of humor you Like, what you Dislike and what you might be too embarrassed to admit ... your Dirty Little Secrets! Put these all together and you have your Laughter IQ.

And remember, it doesn't matter what anyone else thinks about your choices. Your Humor Self-Portrait is not about what's hot on the humor market it's about finding out what kind of humor boosts your own mind and body.

And while your Humor Self-Portrait is all about you, it's still fun to share them as long as people remember not to judge anyone's choices. Sharing charts can be a great bonding experience and a fun connecting tool. So encourage a spouse, a relative, a friend or a colleague to make one, too. You'll find a blank Humor Self-Portrait at the end of the hand-out.

Prescription B: Benefit your Mind and Body With Humor and Laughter

Can giggling boost your immune system? Can a few chuckles help keep your heart healthy? Can humor foster communication, hope and problem solving? The answer to all three of these questions is yes, yes and yes! And that's just a sampling of all the amazing ways humor and laughter can affect your physical and mental wellbeing. However, you don't have to learn every fact. All you really need to know is that humor has such benefits on the mind and body, especially the immune system, the heart and stress levels, that it's time to include it as an important Lifestyle Choice. And guess what? Unlike other Lifestyle Choices, humor will never ask you to combat an addiction or encourage you to get up at six AM to jog. And, it will never expect you to starve yourself! In fact, just the opposite! It's perfectly fine to supersize a chuckle! That's why I call humor The Feel Good Lifestyle.

However, there is one fact that is important to remember. All the positive mental and physical changes can only come from Mirthful Laughter. What's that? Simply put, Mirthful Laughter is humor that leaves one feeling optimistic and relaxed. While Mirthful Laughter may make fun of or point out the weaknesses in our crazy world, it never puts anyone down, creates tension or leaves us with negative feelings. Instead, it offers hope, creates bonds, and helps keep us healthy. Never underestimate the power of mirth!

Prescription C: Coping Humor The Red-Caped Stress Reliever

The Humor Revolution is about laughing more and stressing less. While humor enhances health, stress does the opposite, making the body more vulnerable to disease. Maybe it's time for more of us to stop running around as if we are over caffeinated and in need of a teddy bear to hug! Fortunately, humor can come to the rescue. It can be enjoyed for itself and, it can also offer a way to relieve and diffuse stress. This is called Coping Humor. How does this work? When you smile or laugh, you temporarily distance yourself from a stressful situation. While Coping Humor might not be able to change the situation, it can offer you momentary relief from whatever is troubling or upsetting.

I offer this visual to help you picture how this works: Imagine Coping Humor as a big hook that suddenly descends and lifts you up, up and away from the stress of a situation. Of course, it has to eventually put you back down, but by that time you have hopefully had a chance to breathe deeply, refresh your outlook, and if you are fortunate, return with a new perspective or insight on the problem. While you may not be able to see it, The Humor Hook can be an empowering tool.

Coping Humor can be used for everyday stress and in more difficult circumstances. While this may seem unlikely, be open to the possibility that humor can exist even in the most challenging situations. I remember the last Thanksgiving with my mother at home bedridden with cancer. Knowing how much she loved to cook Thanksgiving dinner, I brought ingredients and pans into her bedroom so she could help. We decided this would make a great special for the food channel and had such fun coming up with titles for the program: Would it be called *The Iron Chief in Bed* or *Thirty Minute Meals in Bed*? Or my favorite: *The Barefoot Contessa in Bed*. She not only laughed she said: "Alice, it's so nice to be with someone who is not afraid to still joke with me."

Prescription D: Developing Your Sense of Humor Using Weapons of Laugh Instruction

Have you ever noticed how funny people are when given the chance? It appears that humor is an innate part of our being that can be developed and nurtured. With that in mind, let's take a look at some simple Weapons of Laugh Instruction you can use to develop your own wit and playfulness.

1. The Truth
While some may not at first see how The Truth can develop humor, I always include it because it's an easy if often overlooked way to add laughs to one's life. All you need to do is activate your Humor Antennae so you can savor the absurdities of everyday life. And they happen all the time, even when you least expect it. Like the time I was at a book fair selling my book: *Where Can I Be Decaffeinated?* Now, this book is nothing more than a collection of funny stories. But that didn't stop a man from rushing up to me to say: "I want to congratulate you! It's about time someone wrote about the evils of caffeine. Are you are planning to single-handedly take on Starbucks and its entire corporation?"

2. Exaggerate

If the truth isn't funny enough, you can always Exaggerate! A trip to a supermarket may not seem amusing until you compare it to climbing Mt. Everest. Hey, don't scoff. Maneuvering through a supermarket can be challenging. You may have to push a shopping cart that only moves sidewise, survive the deadly cold of the frozen food aisle or encounter a canned food avalanche.

3. Surprise!

Surprise can turn an ordinary event or conversation into a laugh-filled moment. I still remember walking through the perfume department of an upscale department store when a woman rushed up to me. I expected a request to douse me with a new expensive perfume being touted by a famous Hollywood actress, but all I saw was a syringe and a needle. I laughed out loud after being asked: "Do you want to hear about our Botox program?"

4. Irony: Isn't Life Strange?

Irony is amusing because it points out the differences in what we expect and what actually does happen. The other day I ran into a parent of a former classmate of my daughter's. The proud daddy told me how his son, a recent graduate in civil engineering was moving east to live and work with two other fellow graduates that between them boasted degrees in electrical and structural engineering. He then added: "All the moms have gone east to help the guys set up house." I cracked up. How funny to think that three young men, who together could build bridges, sky scrapers and electrical plants, still needed their mommies to help them put together a kitchen.

5. Parody

Making fun of existing material is not just for published writers. Anyone who writes anything can use this Weapon of Laugh Instruction. I happen to love making a parody out of a holiday newsletter. Here is an excerpt from one of my favorites:

What a great year we had! Our daughter sold 5,000 boxes of Girl Scout cookies at gunpoint. Our son also worked to raise money for a good cause. His chess team helped raise money for America's War on Obesity by selling five million candy bars. However, my husband may lose his job as Chief of Surgery due to budget cuts. Yet he remains optimistic and has a great alternate plan. If fired, he plans to stand on a street corner with a sign that says: *Will Operate for Food*.

Prescription E: Embracing Humor
So Much Laughter, So Little Time

There are so many ways to increase smiles in your life: activating your Humor Antennae, creating a Humor Self-Portrait and Laugh for the Joy of It. And that's just a few. I have chosen ten other ways to add chuckles to your life. They are listed in no particular order and of course it is up to you to decide which ones you like.

1. Build a Humor Library
Start collecting books, videos, DVD's, whatever tickles you. I like to keep my collection in one place that I call my Humor Library. Every time I need a humor fix, I know just where to go.

2. Create a Funny Bone Boutique
Create, collect or design anything that makes you smile or laugh. In my home we have several including my husband's funny tie collection, a refrigerator door jammed with amusing photos and a computer screen draped with odd-looking chickens. The possibilities are endless!

3. Keep a Humor Journal or a Diary of a Mad Laugher
A humor journal is a wonderful tool because it encourages you to start looking for laughter. It's also fun to be able to read it and relive amusing moments. Where do you start? Keep track of funny street signs, amusing incidences and what you or others do that cracks you up. One of my favorite entries is from my own appointment book. On a Thursday I had written *Dinner with Alice*. I still laugh when I read it. Fortunately, the friend who was having *Dinner with Alice* called to confirm. And who knows where your journal will lead you? Mine turned into a book of amusing tales and spoofs called *Where Can I Be Decaffeinated?*

4. Start a Humor Group or Club
Studies have shown that people with chronic diseases fare better when they participate in a Humor Group, so why not have Humor Groups for everyone? We don't need the excuse of being ill to share funny moments. And a Humor Club can be anything from just sharing amusing moments over tea and cookies to playing games or enjoying a monthly outing to a comedy club. Once again, the possibilities are endless. And, for those of you who don't like joining groups, I have a solution. Start a club of one, you! Take yourself out to a funny event or indulge yourself with a humorous book. The upside to your club is that everyone will get along perfectly.

5. Create a Humor Book Club

Book clubs are popular everywhere these days. So why not start one where people read and share amusing books? Or ask your existing club to set aside a couple of months a year for books that create giggles.

6. Permission to Play

I am giving you permission to start playing because it's important for your health. Do you remember that wonderful saying by an unknown author? *We stop playing because we age and we age because we stop playing.* Try a game of humorous charades, play scrabble with made-up words or host a party where adults break a piñata or play Pin the Tail on the Donkey. Sound silly? I hosted one recently and everyone had the best time.

7. Find a Laugh Partner

It's always wonderful to find that certain someone with whom you love to laugh. How do you find one? I don't have an exact answer but it's amusing to consider a personal ad that might say: *Drop Dead Sexy Laugher seeks same!*

8. Join a Laughter Group and Laugh for the Joy of It

Organized Laughter Groups exist all over the country. Getting together with people to laugh for the sake of laughing can be such fun. You can check the Internet for 'Laughter Clubs' or 'Laughter Yoga' to find out if one exists near you.

9. Become a Member of a Humor or Laughter Organization

There are a number of humor and laughter organizations listed online that anyone can join. Some sponsor laughter clubs, some host conventions, others keep you updated on the latest findings on the power of joy. It's up to you to find the one that's your best fit.

10. Do Whatever Strikes You Funny!

I'm sure that you can come up with many other imaginative ways to embrace humor. I would love to hear how you Humorize your life. You can contact me at:

dralice@laughingwithdralice.com.

"Well," she thought as she finished her reading, "if only all prescriptions were more like A, B, C, D, and E." She particularly enjoyed reading E since Dr. Alice's suggestions were all new to her. Maybe she could even try one of them? They were certainly more appealing than choking down a bowl of *Fiberlicious,* being asphyxiated by the smell of fish oils, stepping on a broken scale, jogging or working out on *The Rack* wearing itchy work out clothes. But what could she do right now? She didn't feel like leaving her house and she didn't have a humor library or a laugh partner yet. It looked like she might have to come up with an imaginative way to embrace humor, but could she do this? She had never really thought of herself as a creative person, especially a comically creative one. So she let out a big sigh and stared into space. But it wasn't space she saw. It was *The Rack* and that's when the idea hit her. "Could I do that?" she wondered? "Or is it too silly?" However, just thinking about it started her laughing. She just had to try it.

She pitter-pattered back to the kitchen, grabbed the box of *Fiberlicious*, the jar of tightly sealed fish oils, some string and a scissors. She then carried this odd assortment back to her bedroom. After laying them down, she went to collect her broken scale, her unused jogging shoes and her scratchy work out clothes. With her collection complete, she began work on her new creation. First she placed the scale underneath *The Rack* where she couldn't use it, but she really didn't need to step on a broken scale anymore, did she? Next, she wrapped her scratchy organic cotton workout clothes made with natural dyes around the pull-up bars. While she had never cared for the reddish brown color on her skin, she had to admit that a little color really jazzed up *The Rack*. She then removed the pair of pricy jogging shoes from their box and tied them to the pull-up bar now wrapped in the workout clothes. They looked terrific hanging there all new and shiny. She was so glad that she had never worn them! Her next job was a bit more complex. She punched a hole in the cereal box with the scissors and threaded it with string. Now *Fiberlicious* was also ready to hang on *The Rack*. And the cereal looked fabulous dangling from the arm curls, plus it was now safely tucked away from her fat-free, calcium-enriched soymilk. Her days of eating glue were finally over. As a final touch, she wrapped string around the neck of the fish oil jar and hung it decoratively above the bench press.

With her masterpiece completed, she stepped back and laughed out loud … again and again. Imagine, after spending all that money on special foods, pills, athletic shoes, a hi-tech scale and a complex piece of exercise equipment, finally, she had found a way to use it that would enhance her health! Just think, every time she walked into her bedroom she would look at her own Weapon of Laugh Instruction and smirk or snicker or titter and that would set off a cascade of positive physical and mental health benefits, wouldn't it? Was this brilliant or what?

Of course, her husband and others might not appreciate her first foray into The Humor Revolution, but that didn't matter, did it? Hadn't Dr. Alice said over and over again: "It's completely up to you to decide how you want to Humorize your life."

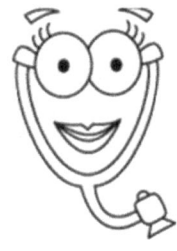

Laughing with Dr. Alice
Experience the Power of Joy

Humor Self-Portrait

Likes   **Dislikes**   **Dirty Little Secrets**

Directions: Under each heading list types of humor or specific people, movies, etc. such as: Stand-up, Slapstick, Wit/Wordplay, Cartoons, Farce, TV Sitcoms, Jokes, Funny Movies, Political Satire, Clowning, Favorite Comedians, British Humor, Comics plus anything you find funny!

Glossary

Dr. Alice's Humor Revolution: How people can actively seek out and use humor and laughter to benefit their minds and bodies and, just as importantly, stop inhaling stress so they can take more pleasure in enjoying life.

Coping Humor: The term used when one draws on humor or laughter to temporarily distance oneself from an upsetting or stressful situation.

Feel Good Lifestyle: Humor is a Feel Good Lifestyle because unlike other Lifestyle Choices, it will never ask you to starve yourself or go jogging at six AM in the cold, dark winter of Los Angeles.

Gelotology: A field of science devoted to studying humor and laughter and how they affect the human body.

Humorize: Anything a person does to add more humor and laughter to their lives.

Humor Antennae: Imaginary antennae that can be activated to remind us that we need to stop and take the time to savor the humorous side of life.

Humorvision: Often there is a choice between seeing stress or humor in a situation. When you choose humor, you are tuning in to Humorvision.

Humor Hook: An imaginary hook that uses humor to temporarily lift you up, up and away from an upsetting circumstance. And while it can't solve a problem, when it sets you back down you may return refreshed with a new outlook on the problem.

Humor Self-Portrait: Is all about you because it's a compilation of all your humor likes and dislikes.

Laugh for the Joy of It: Laughing for the simple joy of experiencing laughter.

Laughs on Learning: Using humor and laughter to facilitate a learning experience.

Laughter IQ: Your IQ is simply everything that you find funny. What it's not is a number!

Lifestyle Choices: Ways that people actively choose to live their lives that can profoundly affect how long their lives will last.

Man-made Stress: A current phenomenon of people voluntarily embracing stress and living their lives as if they are over caffeinated and in need of a teddy bear to hug.

Mirthful Humor/Laughter: A warm-hearted humor or laughter experience that leaves one feeling optimistic and relaxed.

Permission to Play: A reminder to adults that it's still important to play because our bodies thrive on joy and fun. An unknown person said it so well: *We stop playing as we age and we age because we stop playing.*

Psychoneuroimmunology: A field of science that studies the effect of our emotions and behaviors and their connection with the brain and the immune system.

Therapeutic Humor: Using humor and laughter to promote health, wellness and a greater enjoyment of life.

Weapons of Laugh Instruction: There are five Weapons of Laugh Instruction: The Truth, Exaggeration, Surprise, Irony and Parody. Each offers a unique way to develop more humor in your life.

Humor Revolution Reference List

1. Valliant G. *Aging Well: Surprising Guideposts to a Happier Life from the Landmark Harvard Study of Adult Development.* Little, Brown and Co., New York, 2003.
2. Martin GM, et al. Genetic determinants of human health span and life span progress and new opportunities. Plo S Genet. 2007; 3:e125.
3. Fry WF. The physiologic effects of humor, mirth and laughter. JAMA. 1992; 267:1857-8.
4. Godfrey JR. Toward optimal health: The experts discuss therapeutic humor. J Women's Health. 2004; 13:474-479.
5. Fry WF. The biology of humor. Humor. 1994; 7:111-126.
6. Laugh yourself healthy, studies show humor-health link. JAMA News. 2005; 12:1970-1971.
7. Berk L, Tan S, Westengard J. Beta-endorphin and HGH increase are associated with both the anticipation and experience of mirthful laughter. Presented at American Physiological Society session at Experimental Biology 2006, San Fransisco.
8. 8.Weisenberg M, Tepper I, Schwarzwald J. Humor as a cognitive technique for increasing pain tolerance. Pain 1995; 63(2):207-12.
9. Nevo O, Keinan G, Teshimousky-Ardit M. Humor and pain tolerance. Humor. 1993; 6:71.
10. Fried I, Wilson CL, et al. Electric current stimulates laughter. Nature. 1998; 392(6668):650.
11. Shammi P, Stuss DT. Humor appreciation: a role of the right frontal lobe. Brain. 1999; 122(pt 4):657-66.
12. Burchiel RN. Incorporating fun into the business of serious work: the use of humor in group process. Semin Periop Nurs. 1999; 2:60-70.
13. Chauvet S, Hofmeyer A. Humor as a facilitative style in problem based learning environments for nursing students. Nurs Educ Today. 2007; 4:286-92.
14. Isen A. Positive affect facilitates creative problem solving. J Pers Soc Psychol. 1987; 52:1122-1131.
15. Tan SA, Tan LG, Berk LS et al. Mirthful laughter: An effective adjunct therapy in cardiac rehabilitation. Can J Cardiol. 1997; 13(suppl B):190.

16. Clark A, Seider A, Miller M. Inverse association between sense of humor and coronary heart disease. Int J Cardiol. 2001; 80(1):87-88.

17. Miller M, Mangano C, Park Y et al. Laughter and its effect on blood vessels function. Presented at the Scientific Session of the American College of Cardiology, March 7, 2005.

18. Takahashi K, Iwase M, Yamashita K et al. The elevation of natural killer cell activity induced by laughter in a crossover designed study. Int J Molec Med. 2001; 6:646-50.

19. Bennett MP, Zeller JM, Rosenberg L. The effect of mirthful laughter on stress and natural killer cell activity. Altern Ther Health Med. 2003; 9(2):38-45.

20. Berk L, Felten D, Tan S et al. Modulation of neuroimmune parameters during the eustress of humor associated with mirthful laughter. Altern Ther Health Med. 2001; 7(2):74-6.

21. Palesh O, Butler LD, Kooopman C et al. Stress history and breast cancer recurrence. J Psychosom Res. 2007; 63(3):233-239.

22. McClelland D, Cheriff AD. The immunoenhancing effects of humor on secretory IgA and resistance to respiratory infections. Psychol and Health. 1997; 12:329-44.

23. Perara S et al. Increases in salivary lysozyme and IgA concentrations and secretory rates independent of salivary flow rates following viewing of a humorous videotape. Int J of Behav Med. 1998; 5:118-128.

24. Rice EL. Wellness/problem patient. Audio-Digest Family Practice. 2007; 55(45).

25. Selye H. *The Stress of Life.* McGraw Hill, New York, 1956.

26. Cousins N. *Anatomy of an Illness.* WW Norton and CO, New York, 1979.

27. Cousins N. *Head First: The Biology of Hope.* Dutton, New York, 1989.

28. Weisiger R. Gastroenterology for the internist. Audio-Digest Internal Medicine. 2007; 54(6).

29. Ader R, Felten DL, Cohen N. *Psychoneuroimmunology.* Academic Press, San Diego, 1991.

30. Foley E, Matheis R, Schaefer C. Effect of forced laughter on mood. Psychol Rep. 2002; 90(1):14-25.

31. Levenson R, Ekman P, Friesen W. Voluntary facial actions generates emotion-specific autonomic nervous system activity. Psychophysiology. 1990; 27:363-384.

32. Soussignan B. Duchenne smile, emotional experience and autonomic reactivity: a test of the facial feedback hypothesis. Emotion. 2002; 2(1):52-74.

33. Ekman P, Davidson R. The brain behind that happy face. Science. 1993; 264(5159):644

34. Kataria M. *Laugh for No Reason*. Madhuri International, Mumbai, 1999.

Note to Reader: Hundreds of scientific papers have been published on the mental and physical effects of humor and laughter on the body. This is a representative list, not an exhaustive one. For more studies type in PubMed on your favorite search engine. Once there, any topic of interest can be easily accessed.

978-0-595-49536-8
0-595-49536-2